Dear Cherise,

With every
good wish for
happiness and
good health!

Elaine
Nussba[...]

Recovery

RECOVERY

From Cancer to Health
Through Macrobiotics

By Elaine Nussbaum

Japan Publications, Inc.

Note to the reader: This book is not a substitute for professional medical care. It is essential that any reader who has a serious illness consult with their physician before implementing the approach to health outlined in this book.

Published by Japan Publications, Inc., Tokyo & New York

Distributors:
United States: *Kodansha International/USA, Ltd., through Harper & Row, Publishers, Inc., 10 East 53rd Street, New York, N. Y. 10022.* South America: *Harper & Row, Publishers, Inc., International Department.* Canada: *Fitzhenry & Whiteside Ltd., 195 Allstate Parkway, Markham, Ontario, L3R 4T8.* Mexico & Central America: *HARLA S. A. de C. V. Apartado 30–546, Mexico 4, D. F.* British Isles: *International Book Distributors Ltd., 66 Wood Lane End, Hemel Hempstead, Herts HP2 4RG.* European Continent: *Fleetbooks, S. A., c/o Feffer and Simons (Nederland) B. V., Rijnkade 170, 1382 GT Weesp, The Netherlands.* Australia & New Zealand: *Bookwise International, 1 Jeanes Street, Beverley, South Australia 5007.* The Far East & Japan: *Japan Publications Trading Co., Ltd., 1–2–1, Sarugaku-cho, Chiyoda-ku, Tokyo 101.*

First edition: May 1986

LCCC No. 85–081364
ISBN 0–87040–643–4

Printed in U.S.A.

To my husband Ralph,
my parents, my children,
and my sisters,
whose love and support have sustained me
through sickness and health.

Foreword

When I first heard Elaine Nussbaum's account of her experience with widespread metastatic cancer, I was overwhelmed. I found it difficult to believe that anyone could have endured what Elaine endured and have survived so well, both physically and emotionally. I had known Elaine for several months socially and had always been impressed by her warm, outgoing, friendly, and energetic personality. It was not until we were both attending the same conference and Elaine spoke about her condition that I learned of her ordeal. I sat in the audience spellbound. I felt as though I had stopped breathing as I listened to insult after insult her body had taken, finding it hard to believe that any one person could go through all of that and come out in what appeared to be a better condition.

I have been a Board Certified Family Practitioner practicing medicine for over twenty-five years, and I must admit that Elaine's story is the most amazing account of healing that I have ever encountered. As I sat in the audience I felt myself profoundly moved, both by the woman telling her story and by the marvelous ability of the human body and spirit to overcome seemingly impossible difficulties.

Given the medical history of her illness, Elaine's astonishing recovery and the quality of her life demand that we in the medical profession look more closely at this approach to healing and to the accounts of others like her who have used macrobiotics to recover from serious illness. I have been impressed by patients I have met who have decided to practice macrobiotics for various conditions. From my experience with them and the macrobiotic approach, I can certainly attest to the fact that macrobiotics promotes good health and is a definite contributing factor in the recovery from disease.

Macrobiotics has its roots in the very ancient philosophy of harmonizing with nature through the balancing of complementary opposites. In the Far East, these were known as yin and yang. I am very respectful of a traditional discipline that has contributed so much to the health of culture and civilization for so many thousands of years and feel that we as modern medical practitioners, and our patients, would benefit greatly from opening our minds to this way of promoting health, and preventing and relieving disease.

MARTHA C. COTTRELL, M.D.
New York, N.Y.

Preface

Falling in love was the real thing for Elaine and me in 1954. While the sideline gossipers and para-statisticians predicted that our young marriage in 1957 would not last, we defied their odds and established a lasting union based on the twin pillars of deep love and total commitment. Having shared most of my life with her, Elaine's story is also my story, and her recovery is one of the highlights of my life.

Until she was eighteen, Elaine experienced few hardships as she grew up in a close family blessed with good health. This environment was probably responsible for her warm, happy, radiant and care-free disposition. For the next nineteen years following our marriage, Elaine devoted herself to being wife and mother. She genuinely enjoyed her role, and in a natural and innate manner, played the major part in raising our four children.

In 1976, after our youngest child began school, Elaine decided to go to college to prepare herself for the next phase in our lives. She now, for the first time, had to take on more than could easily fit into a normal day without sacrificing what she regarded as her continuing household responsibilities.

In 1979, I added a real burden when I broke the news that my employer had asked me to relocate from New Jersey to California. It was a difficult decision for all of us, but most especially for Elaine, who was torn between my desire to move the family cross-country and the children's wishes to remain on the East Coast.

It is very likely that the stress, tension, and pressure which

Elaine experienced during these years contributed to her declining health.

When Elaine was diagnosed as having cancer in 1980, her biological immune system had obviously failed, and as time would tell, her body was to experience a metastasis that would threaten her life. While standard and advanced medical procedures kept her alive for several years and reduced the intolerable pain associated with the spread of cancer in the spine, it was Elaine's understanding and belief in natural nutrition, combined with her strong determination to live, that finally saved her life.

Having had a scientific training, I was admittedly a skeptic early in 1983 when Elaine decided to adopt an alternative approach based on a strange diet. While I agreed to be supportive, seeing that Elaine was so determined and had not given up her fight to live, I did not share her faith that diet without medication could restore her health.

Elaine's story, which follows, has revolutionized my beliefs, and I hope it will inspire many readers who might derive benefit from the macrobiotic approach.

RALPH NUSSBAUM

Acknowledgments

I would like to thank all the people who helped bring this book into being: Michio Kushi, who suggested that I write it; Edward Esko, Alex Jack, Sherman Goldman, Stevan Goldin and Phillip Janetta for their editorial assistance; and Debra Nussbaum, for her advice and guidance in editing the final draft.

I am grateful to my husband Ralph and my sister Phyllis Goldschmidt who read and reread my manuscript and who were unhesitatingly generous with their time and advice. My gratitude also goes to Dr. Justin Bergman for reviewing and deciphering my medical records and for encouraging me to write this book.

I would like to express my endless appreciation to my macrobiotic teachers and advisors—Michio Kushi, Shizuko Yamamoto, Murray Snyder, Denny Waxman, and Bill Spear— for their teachings, writings, lectures, dietary recommendations, and lifestyle suggestions that have enabled me to better understand the macrobiotic way of life.

Part I

"If we leave Nature alone, she recovers gently
from the disorder into which she has fallen.
It is our anxiety, our impatience, which spoils
all; and nearly all men die of their remedies,
not of their diseases."

—MOLIERE

Chapter 1

CONSCIOUSNESS RETURNED SLOWLY. I opened my eyes and looked up at the dull white ceiling. I tried to turn my head—it didn't move. My eyes closed again and I dozed. A form appeared next to my stretcher and wrapped something around my arm. Blood pressure. My wrist was being squeezed. Pulse. I opened my eyes again. Something was being taken off my face. Tubes from my nostrils. I turned my head.

The room was crowded with stretchers. They were not lined up in rows, but scattered around haphazardly. On each stretcher lay a person, encased in white sheets. Bandaged heads, bandaged arms, and bandaged feet extended from the white sheets. Nurses were bustling around, taking pulses, adjusting tubes, administering medications.

Memory began to return. I had entered the hospital that morning, April 16, 1980, for what I had thought would be a routine dilation and curettage. For the past eleven months, I had been having long and excessive menstrual periods. I had bled to the point of becoming severely anemic. Repeated Pap smears and pelvic examinations showed nothing. Today's D&C was an attempt to determine the cause.

From my stretcher in the recovery room I could see the big swinging doors. Constant movement—doors opening and closing continuously, stretchers being moved out, new ones being brought in. My eyes focused on a blackboard hanging adjacent to the swinging doors. In bold letters was printed, **"Hold Till One O'Clock."** Under the heading was one name —NUSSBAUM.

A nurse appeared again to take my pulse and blood pressure.

"Am I all right?" I asked hesitantly.

"Fine," she answered.

"Why am I being held till one o'clock?" I asked.

"Those were your doctor's orders," was her reply.

"Do you know why?" I continued.

"No," she said, while she marked down my vital signs. And then she disappeared.

I closed my eyes and dozed again. My stretcher began to move. I was being pushed towards the big swinging doors. Out of the recovery room and down the hospital corridors I rode, until we reached my semi-private room. My husband Ralph was waiting in the doorway. He looked white—whiter than the sheets that were encasing me.

"Hi hon," I mumbled as my stretcher turned into the room and was positioned next to the inside bed.

I was lifted from the stretcher onto the bed and covered with a new set of white sheets. Ralph came in, planted a kiss on my forehead, and took my hand. I looked up at him. Pale as a ghost he stood there, trying to manage a weak smile.

"I'm okay, hon," I whispered. "Really, I'm fine."

He squeezed my hand. "This is worse for him than it is for me," I thought.

My doctor appeared. He came around to the other side of my bed and sat down. The room was quiet; no one was there but the three of us. I looked up at the doctor questioningly, not expecting to hear anything dramatic or profound.

"I have bad news and I have good news," he said slowly and deliberately. "The bad news is that we found a tumor in your uterus—and it is malignant. The good news is that we can treat it."

Silence. I lay there staring at him, dumbfounded. What was he saying? Ralph sqeezed my hand again.

"Don't worry, Lainzie," he said. "We're in this together. Whatever happens now, we'll both fight it together."

* * *

Malignant tumor. Cancer. Treatments. My doctor was telling me that I had cancer. I tried to listen to what he was saying. He had not performed the dilation and curettage. The tumor was too large and he had not wanted to scrape or disturb it at all for fear that it might spread. He had collected some surrounding cells and had sent them to the laboratory to be analyzed. We would know the results in two days.

I was listening to a story. This wasn't happening to me. Cancer was something that happened to other people; one read about it in the newspaper or heard about it on the radio. People were dying of cancer every day—other people— strangers. Not me.

"Will I need surgery?" I asked the doctor. I was talking about someone else. I was being objective and I felt nothing.

"Yes," he answered. "You'll need surgery."

"When will you operate?" I asked.

"Probably in three or four months," he answered.

"Three or four months!" I nearly shouted, "three or four months—Why? I don't want it for three or four months. Why can't you take it out now?"

"It's too large," he answered gently. "If we remove it now, it will spread for sure."

He went on to explain that it would be much better to shrink the tumor before trying to remove it. This could be accomplished with radiation. Daily radiation treatments, possibly followed by a radium implant, would cause the tumor to shrivel up and die. "We have had success with this mode of treatment," he said. "Sometimes the tumor becomes so small that by the time of the surgery it is barely visible." This is what he was hoping for in my case.

What followed was a barrage of questions. What kind of tumor do I have? Exactly where is it? How come the Pap smears didn't pick it up? What kind of radiation will I get? How many treatments? How will you know if the radiation is effective? Suppose it's not? Could the tumor possibly shrink and disappear so that I won't need the surgery? Will I need chemotherapy? Will my hair fall out? Can I go home this afternoon?"

The doctor listened patiently. I would probably need about twenty radiation treatments, he said, and he did not think I would need chemotherapy. However, nothing could be decided for sure until we received the pathology report on the tumor. It was now Wednesday—we would know on Friday.

I could not leave the hospital. Between today and Friday he wanted to run some tests to be sure that the cancer hadn't spread outside of the uterus. Today I would just rest. Thursday and Friday we would schedule a chest X-ray, a liver scan, a barium enema, an intravenous pylogram, an ultrasound scan of the pelvis, and a bone scan. I could plan to go home on Friday evening.

I did not want to just rest. I was too agitated, and besides, I wanted to get out of the hospital as soon as possible.

"Could we do the tests today and tommorrow?" I asked. "Then maybe I could go home tommorow night?"

The doctor didn't want me to leave before Friday, but he would try to schedule one or two tests for this afternoon or evening.

Promising to let us know as soon as he made some arrangements, he left the room. Ralph and I were alone. Ralph sat down on the bed, still holding my hand. He squeezed again. The floodgates opened, and finally, we cried.

* * *

"Why me?" I wondered. I had always enjoyed good health. As a child, I had never been in a hospital, and as an adult, only for the birth of each of my four children. My parents, now in their late sixties and early seventies, were well, and my two younger sisters and their children also enjoyed good health. Except for my grandfather, who died of esophageal cancer at the age of eighty-four, there was no history of cancer, or any other degenerative disease, in my family.

Religion had always played an important part in my life. I observed the Sabbath and the Jewish holidays, and I attended Synagogue regularly. Why was this happening to me? I had always tried to be a good person. I was giving and caring, a devoted daughter, sister, wife, mother, and friend. Only when my youngest child had started first grade did I begin to do something outside my home—to go back to college. My tastes and style were basically natural; I dressed simply, and wore very little makeup. I ate well, retired early, and did not smoke or drink. Now, only one month away from college graduation. . . . Why cancer? Why now? Why me?

* * *

A liver scan was to be my first test, and it was scheduled for that very afternoon. When the nurse arrived with a wheelchair, I was a little scared but ready to begin. I was wheeled to the nuclear medicine department where I joined the mass of patients on stretchers, in wheelchairs, and on rows of long wooden benches awaiting their turn with the scanning machine. On line, I was injected with a radioactive dye; it would take approximately twenty minutes for the dye to settle in my spleen and liver.

Three technicians greeted me in the scanning room, and one of them described the procedure. I would be scanned from a number of positions; standing up with my midsection pressed against the machine as in a hug, lying on my back, lying on one side, then on my stomach, and finally lying on my other side. The procedure would be painless, and I could just relax.

I was helped out of the wheelchair and butted up against the machine. I had hugged many people in my life, but never a cold, monstrous machine. I shuddered, closed my eyes, and the scanner was switched on.

My legs began to weaken, and I felt an overwhelming desire to keep my eyes closed and lie down and sleep. Instead, I opened my eyes, and turning my head slightly to the right, I could see a screen with the shape of a liver clearly displayed on it. On the liver was an array of tiny dots, blinking on and off like a movie theater marquee.

"Is that my liver?" I asked to no one in particular.

"That's your liver," came a reply from behind me.

Nausea overtook me, and my legs turned to water.

"I'm going down," I mumbled, and my head started spinning as I lost my grip on the machine.

I lay flat on the floor. A cool towel was on my forehead.

"She's coming to," a voice above me said, and I opened my eyes to see four people staring down at me.

"You fainted," said one of them, and they helped me up and back into the wheelchair.

"You're very weak," I was told. "We'll send you back to your room and reschedule you for another time."

"No!" I objected. "I feel better now, I'm fine. Please let me try again. I know I can do it."

Fear was welling up inside me. I wanted to get out of there fast, but I certainly did not want to have to come back. Suppose they couldn't reschedule me for a few days—I was determined to go home on Friday.

"Please," I begged, practically in tears. "Please let me try again."

They looked at each other, seemingly confused.

"Okay," someone said finally. "Let's try it lying down first."

I was helped onto the table where I made a concentrated effort not to look at the screen. Afterwards, in the hugging position, I kept my eyes closed the entire time.

When the procedure was over, I asked timidly, "Does it show anything?"

"Your doctor will tell you the results," someone answered.

I searched their faces for some kind of clue, but I could

detect nothing. Finally, I was wheeled back to my room where Ralph was waiting for me in the doorway.

Was it still Wednesday? So much had happened since I checked into the hospital that morning. And tomorrow would be another full day. I was scheduled for chest X-rays to check my lungs, a barium enema for my colon, an intravenous pylogram for my kidneys, a bone scan, and an ultrasound scan to check my entire pelvic area. Testing would begin in the morning and finish in the late afternoon. I had every intention of leaving the hospital on Friday and spending the weekend at home with my family. But now, Ralph would have to leave and break the news to the children. He would also call my parents, his mother, and my two sisters. I did not envy him this task.

* * *

Ralph and I had been married almost twenty-three years, and we had four children. Debra was twenty-one, a senior in college; Rachel was nineteen, a sophomore in college; and Rhonda was fifteen, a sophomore in high school. Our son Jeffrey was only ten, a fifth grader. I worried about the children. How would this affect them? Would Debra and Rachel have to drop out of college to help care for me? Would Rhonda's teenage years be marred by her mother's cancer? Would she be embarrassed and ashamed? Would her friends still come? Would Jeffrey understand? A teacher in his school had recently died from cancer. Would he think I was going to die too? Would his friends on the schoolbus tell him that cancer means death? Would he have nightmares? How much of my children's time would be spent worrying about me—and about themselves? Would they feel vulnerable? What kind of youth would they have?

What would this do to my parents? What could be worse for parents than to watch a child suffer? May parents were retired and living in Florida. They visited us often, we visited with them, and we spoke on the phone regularly. They were so proud of their family: their three daughters and sons-in-law and their twelve grandchildren—all happy, healthy, close, celebrating the holidays and family occasions together. What would this cancer do to them?

Shayndee and Phyllis had been more than my sisters; they were my best friends. We had shared so much—our childhood, our school compositions, our clothes, our dating experiences, the birth of our children and the joys and problems of raising them, luncheons alone, dinners with our husbands, favorite recipes, and bridge games. Now this. Shayndee and Phyllis would be devastated.

Poor Ralph. Not only would he have to deal with my cancer and his own emotions, he would have to hold the whole family together. What had Ralph ever done to deserve this? Ralph was a special person—a good son and brother, a wonderful husband and father. Though his job required some traveling, he was always around when we needed him. Together we had changed diapers, helped with homework, and driven carpools. It was always a treat for the children, and for me, when Ralph cooked supper on Sunday nights. For many summers, we had rented a cabin on a lake and spent wonderful family vacations together. We had saved and planned for our future. We had built a marriage, a home, and a close family. I loved Ralph. I did not want to cause him this anguish.

Guilt. I was spoiling life for my family. From happy and confident, they would become saddened, worried, and fearful. They would become helpless; what could they do to ease my suffering—and their own? Nothing. Suppose I died? There would be sadness forever, at every Sabbath, at every birthday, Bar-Mitzvah, and wedding. Anger. Anger at the cancer. How could this happen to me? Anger at God. How could He allow this to happen? How could He destroy my family?

*   *   *

Thursday's breakfast was the same as my evening snack the night before—a laxative. I would be all cleaned out for a full day of tests. My first appointment was for chest X-rays. I was wheeled to the X-ray room where an energetic technician positioned me at the machine, retreated into a shielded booth, called "Hold your breath," and clicked a shot. He then appeared at my side, positioned me for the next exposure, and ran back to his safety booth to shoot the next pose. This routine continued until the required number of pictures had been taken.

My next appointment was for an intravenous pylogram. The technician explained the procedure. Dye would be injected into an arm vein. The dye would outline my kidneys and bladder, and pictures would be taken.

I lay on the table under the machine and submitted to the injection.

The reaction was immediate. Within seconds, I felt an intense heat rushing through my body. Warm liquid raced through my abdomen, my genital area, and down to the tips of my toes. Then up, swirling around and around through my head.

"I'm going to faint," I mumbled.

"You'll be all right," said the technician. "Just close your eyes and rest. You'll feel better in a few minutes."

The sensation soon passed, my body relaxed, and I started to cry.

The technician came over to my side.

"What's the matter?" she asked gently. "Are you having any pain?"

"No," I sobbed. "I'm just so scared."

"What are you afraid of?" she asked, handing me a tissue. "This won't hurt you; it won't even be uncomfortable any more." She put her hand over mine and I cried harder.

"I have cancer," I said between sobs. "I just found out

yesterday, and today I'm having all these tests, and I'm just so scared that they're going to find something."

She took my used tissue and gave me a clean one. I wiped my eyes and then cried some more. She patted my arm. I couldn't stop the tears.

"I have a husband and four children," I sobbed. "I don't want to die."

"Maybe you won't," she said gently. "Try not to worry. Everything will probably be fine."

She explained the breathing procedure, and I held my breath while she took the necessary pictures. Then she helped me back into my wheelchair. As an orderly appeared to wheel me away, I thanked the technician for being so kind to me. I would be kind too, I decided. If I would be good and be nice to the doctors and technicians, I thought, maybe they wouldn't find anything.

Back in my wheelchair, I was pushed along for my next appointment—a barium enema. There was a long wait for this procedure; wheelchairs were lined up in a row against the wall and a doctor was going from one patient to the next administering injections.

"Why do I need an injection for a barium enema?" I asked.

"The injection is not for the enema," I was told. "It's for your bone scan."

"But I'm not getting a bone scan now," I argued.

He checked my chart. "You're scheduled for a bone scan later on," he said, "and I have to give you the injection now because there must be a three hour wait between the injection and the scan."

"Won't it interfere with the barium I'm having in the meantime?" I asked.

"No," he answered, and before I could ask another question, I was injected.

My turn finally came. Barium was given and pictures were taken. It was not as unpleasant as I thought it would be.

My last test for the day was the bone scan. Again I sat in

line. Between the wheelchairs and stretchers ahead of me, people had pulled up chairs and were reading magazines. I estimated that there would be a long wait, and I was upset. I had thought my appointment meant that I had a special time reserved. By the time my turn arrived, I was exhausted. Once again I was put on a table under a big machine. I lay on my back, absolutely still. The machine would be lowered very close to my body, I was told. It would start at the top of my head, move slowly, and scan me to the tips of my toes. Then, it would turn under the foot of the table and move upwards until it would come back to my head. I could just relax. I did better than that. As soon as the machine was clicked on, I closed my eyes and fell asleep.

Back in my room, dinner was waiting. Hospital food, I was learning, was not a gourmet's delight. It's good that I'm going home tomorrow, I thought. Otherwise I would have to ask Ralph to bring me some decent food.

The phone rang. It was my sister Phyllis.

"Is it okay if I come?" she asked.

"You don't have to come, Phyl," I answered. "It's really not necessary."

Phyllis lived with her husband Dave and their four children in Teaneck, New Jersey, a forty minute drive from our home in West Orange and about fifty minutes from the hospital. She was calling from work. She had been calling Ralph all day, and now that he told her that the tests for the day were completed and I was back in my room, she wanted to see me. She would leave work early and come straight to the hospital. Dave would come home and take care of the children. Not wanting her to be bothered with all these arrangements, not wanting to impose on Dave and the children, I told her not to come. Phyllis was confused. How could I not want her to be with me?

"I won't come if you don't want me to," she said. "But if you just want to save me the time and effort, don't. I really want to come."

"Well hurry up," I told her, suddenly so happy that she was coming. "Come right now. I'm only going to be here until tomorrow."

Phyllis arrived, and Ralph, who had been in the hospital all day, left. He came back in the evening with our four children.

I thought I looked okay. I had brushed my hair and put on some lipstick. I had straightened out the sheets and cranked the bed up to a sitting position. I wanted so much to look good to the children; I didn't want them to worry. I thought I was convincing. They said I looked good; they thought I looked awful.

Debra and Rachel understood the seriousness of the situation. If we were lucky, radiation would shrink the tumor, it would be removed, and I would be fine. But what if there was involvement in other organs? What might lie ahead? And the fear—fear of the unknown; they were dealing with the same fear as Ralph and I were, and they were hurting.

Rhonda had not fully accepted the idea that her mother had cancer. People with cancer were sick; they looked sick, they acted sick, and other people took care of them. Her mother was fine. Just yesterday morning, like every other morning, hadn't I prepared breakfast, packed lunch, and said, "Have a good day," as the schoolbus pulled up? How could I have cancer?

We weren't sure about how much to tell Jeffrey—he was only ten years old. We decided not to use the word "cancer" just yet. Ralph told him that I had a tumor, a growth, that would have to come out, and that I would need an operation in a few months. This would suffice, we agreed, until the weekend, when I would be back home and up-and-about. So Jeffrey gave me a quick kiss in the hospital and turned his attention to the new things he was seeing for the first time— beds that went up and down, intravenous equipment, medicines and bandages in all shapes and sizes, and a TV that could be turned on and off from the bed.

The family left, and I was alone—alone with my thoughts. What would the tests show? Was there cancer in my lungs, my liver, my kidneys, my bones? Tomorrow morning the doctor would come to tell me whether I would live or die. I couldn't sleep. Thoughts kept popping in and out of my head. Would I have a lot of pain? How long would I suffer? Would my family come to wish for my death? How long would I live? Months? Weeks? My imagination was running wild. I pictured my funeral. I was in the box, dead, and everyone was crying. I was being irrational, I told myself. The tests would show that there was no spread, and I would be fine. Hundreds of people had tumors removed and went on to lead perfectly normal lives. But I couldn't convince myself. I couldn't sleep.

By six-thirty Friday morning, Ralph was at the hospital. The doctor arrived shortly before seven. My chest X-rays and my liver scan were negative. Relief. He didn't have the results of the other tests yet. He would go to check and let us know. A half hour later he was back. Barium enema, negative. Intravenous pylogram, negative. The bone scan results hadn't come back yet. Relief turned to panic. Why weren't the results in? How long does it take to read a bone scan? Maybe they just didn't want to tell me. Maybe I had cancer in my bones. Which bones? My bones felt fine. Besides, I always ate cottage cheese and yogurt for calcium. My heart was pounding, and I was sweating profusely.

"When will we know?" I asked the doctor.

"I'll be in the hospital all morning," he said. "As soon as I know, I'll be back to tell you."

A nurse appeared with two turquoise pitchers of water and a matching plastic cup.

"Mrs. Nussbaum?" she asked, coming over to my bed.

I nodded.

"You'll have to drink all this water," she said. "You must not urinate. The ultrasound scan must be done when you have a full bladder. When you have to go so badly that you can't hold it any more, ring for a nurse and someone will come to bring you upstairs for the tests."

"All this water?" I asked with disbelief.

"It's eight cups," she said. "Usually that's enough, but you may need more." She turned to leave. "Remember," she called back, "do not urinate, no matter how strong the urge."

Ralph and I looked at the two full pitchers. He poured some water into the turquoise cup and handed it to me.

"Drink some," he said.

"I can't," I answered. "I'm not thirsty. Besides, I have to go to the bathroom."

Suddenly the urge to urinate became strong. And I hadn't had a single sip yet. Ralph handed me the cup again. I could not drink any. I never drank plain water. I didn't like it. I drank Postum or tea with a little milk in it. Occasionally I would have some fruit juice. But never plain water.

Ralph went out to find a nurse and tell her I couldn't drink the water. He reappeared with two forty-six ounce cans of fruit juice—one apple juice and one orange juice.

"Didn't they have any apricot nectar?" I asked.

Ralph left again to get some apricot nectar. Now we had three big cans of juice. And no can opener. Ralph left again and came back with a can opener. He poured me some apricot nectar, and I started sipping.

When I couldn't drink another drop and I felt that I was ready to explode, we rang for the nurse. She looked at the two full pitchers of water, and the two-and-a-half cans of juice. We should have poured some down the drain, I thought.

"You didn't drink enough," said the nurse.

"Yes, I did," I said. "I can't drink any more. And I really need a bathroom desperately."

"Your bladder is not full enough," she responded. "You'll have to drink some more."

As soon as she left, Ralph poured most of the water down the drain. We waited a few minutes and rang again.

"I'm ready," I announced as soon as a different nurse

appeared in the doorway. "I'm more than ready. I don't think
I can make it from the bed to the wheelchair."

"Hold it in," said the nurse. "I'll get you upstairs as fast
as I can."

Someone else was having an ultrasound scan, and I had
to wait It was not more than ten minutes, but it felt like ten
hours. Finally my turn came. I was helped onto a table,
and a technician moved an instrument across by belly. On the
side of the table was a screen, and projected on the screen
was my bladder. I remembered my liver scan, and I looked
the other way.

"Your bladder's not full enough," said the technician.
"We'll wait about half an hour and try again. In the meantime, you can drink some more."

"Oh, no," I pleaded. "I can't wait another second." I was
getting panicky. "If I move an inch," I said, "I'll surely
urinate all over the table."

I crossed my legs. I was trying desperately to keep my
hands away from my crotch.

"You've got to do it now," I insisted.

"We'll try," he said, seeing my agony.

He resumed moving his instrument around my mid-section.
I prayed that it wouldn't be a long procedure—I knew I
couldn't control myself much longer. Finally it was over, and
a nurse came to help me take the few steps to the bathroom.

Back in my room, Ralph was waiting. Before I had a
chance to tell him about my adventure upstairs, my doctor
walked into the room. One look at his ashen face told me that
something was wrong.

* * *

The pathology on my tumor had been completed. I did not
have the common uterine carcinoma. What I had was a mixed
tumor—a carcinosarcoma that was embedded in the muscle
of the connective tissue in the lining of the uterus. This was

a rare tumor, the kind that a doctor sees once in twenty years, and then usually in a woman over seventy. A virulent tumor—one that would need to be treated aggressively.

My doctor, an obstetrician gynecologist, had decided to call in a specialist He was recommending a top doctor, a gynecological oncologist, whose expertise was in treating female cancers. She was a well-known and highly sought-after oncologist, and she had an office in the hospital I was now in. He had set up an appointment for late that same morning, and he would accompany us on our first meeting with her.

My heart was pounding, my throat felt tight, and whatever strength I had left was being sapped from my body. What did he mean by "a rare tumor?" Why was it too complicated for him? I didn't want another doctor. I just wanted to go home. He had promised I could go home today. Why did I have a virulent tumor? What makes a tumor virulent anyway? Maybe he was wrong. I choked on my question, "Will I need chemotherapy?"

"You probably will," he answered. "The oncologist will decide on the treatment, and she probably will recommend some chemotherapy."

My tear-filled eyes were running over. I dabbed at them with the sleeve of my bathrobe.

"Will my hair fall out?" I whispered.

He came over to my wheelchair, put his arm around me, and squeezed my shoulder.

"It might not," he said kindly. "Not everyone who has chemotherapy loses their hair. And if it does fall out," he continued, "it will grow in just as beautiful as it is now."

I was crying uncontrollably. I looked up at Ralph, pale and helpless as he stood over me handing me tissue after tissue and trying to console me. "Help me," I pleaded silently. "Take me out of here." I didn't want a rare tumor. I didn't want any tumor. I didn't want to have cancer. I just wanted to go home.

Ralph looked from me to the doctor, helplessly.

"Let her cry," the doctor said. "It's okay for her to cry. It's a perfectly normal reaction."

And promising to meet us later at the oncologist's office, he left us alone with our misery.

* * *

I sat in my wheelchair in the oncologist's office. Against the wall to my right was a file cabinet and a desk with a phone on it. On the wall, above the desk, was a big picture of a mother tiger and her baby. To my left was a row of multi-colored chairs, broken up by a table with a pile of magazines. On the wall, another picture of a tiger. My doctor sat on one of the chairs. Ralph paced back and forth between us. We waited for the oncologist.

She walked in briskly, smiled, and introduced herself. I watched her pick up my folder and glance through it. She seemed so efficient and so professional, both in her dress and in her mannerisms. She spoke rapidly with a foreign accent, and it was difficult for me to understand her. We listened intently as she spoke.

Somewhere in the middle of the biological explanations, my mind wandered, but it returned quickly when the course of my treatment was being explained. I would have to begin chemotherapy immediately: this Monday morning and for the following four days I would be given four hundred milligrams of Cytoxan intravenously. I would have a week to rest, then I would begin radiation treatments, every day for four or five weeks. Depending on my condition after the radiation, I might need a radium implant. She would determine this with my radiotherapist when the time came. I would then have a few weeks to recover from the treatments and to build myself up for the surgery, which would probably be some time in August. Beginning now, throughout the radiation and up until the time of the surgery, I would take chemotherapy orally: Cytoxan and Megace three times a day.

"This is a very aggressive tumor," she told us, "so we will have to treat it aggressively."

I was crying again. Was this really happening to me? This was serious business now—chemotherapy, radiation, surgery. I had felt fine until two days ago when I checked into the hospital for what I thought was going to be a routine dilation and curettage. What was I getting involved in? I didn't want any part of this drama. I just wanted to go home.

"Can I take her home now?" Ralph was asking the oncologist.

"It would be better for her to stay and have the chemotherapy as an inpatient," she replied.

I stared at her. Self-pity was turning to anger. I didn't like this woman. She was so efficient, so knowledgeable, so in control. She was taking charge of my life, and I would have to do as she said. And she wanted to keep me in the hospital.

"Why would it be better to keep her as an inpatient?" Ralph asked.

There were a few reasons. One was that it was uncertain how I would react to the chemotherapy. Side effects could be severe, and if I were in the hospital I could be watched and taken care of. I would be tired and weak, and staying in the hospital would eliminate the daily back and forth trips for the treatments. Another consideration was financial. Most insurance policies covered chemotherapy for inpatients. But for outpatients coverage was usually only partial.

Ralph asked about the cost, and I nearly fell out of my wheelchair when she answered. This was getting ridiculous.

Maybe I should stay, I started to think, suppressing my mounting rage and trying to be practical. Suppose I would be very sick? Who would take care of me? The fear was coming back. How would I get to the hospital every day? Ralph couldn't just take another week off from work. Maybe someone else could take me. I didn't want anyone else. And what about the cost? There was no way we could afford to pay for this. I felt I should agree to stay, but I didn't want to stay. I desperately wanted to go home.

"Maybe I should stay," I said to Ralph, trying to sound brave. I was choking back the oncoming tears.

Ralph looked from me to the oncologist.

"We don't live so far from the hospital," he said. "I can bring her every day, and if she gets sick, I'll take care of her. I don't care about the money. I want to bring her home."

I looked at the oncologist hopefully. She smiled slightly as she nodded in agreement, and I felt my body go limp with relief. She wanted to build up my blood before starting the chemotherapy, so she would schedule two blood transfusions for this afternoon. I could leave in the early evening.

My tears flowed freely. I was going home.

* * *

I did not go home on Friday. Or on Saturday. I had an unexpected reaction to the second blood transfusion.

The first transfusion was uneventful. About an hour into the second one, I noticed that my arm was red and swollen around the injection site.

"Look at my arm," I said to Ralph. "Do you think we should call a nurse?"

Ralph rang for a nurse. None appeared. The circle on my arm seemed to be growing wider.

"Look," I said to Ralph. "It's red and white, all splotchy."

Ralph pressed the button again for a nurse. The splotches were traveling down my arm towards my wrist, and up towards my shoulder. Now red and white welts were spreading around my neck and up onto my face. Ralph ran out of the room, grabbed the first nurse he saw, and pulled her in to look at me. She immediately disconnected my tubing, told me not to move, and ran out to get the head nurse. Ralph and I watched, horrified, as the welts emerged on my chest, abdomen, and thighs. When the head nurse arrived, I was in full bloom, covered from head to toe with red and white splotchy welts.

"It's a reaction," the nurse said. "It happens sometimes," and she plunged a long needle into my buttock.

"What's that for?" I asked.

"To take away the reaction. I'll call your doctor."

My oncologist had a whole team of interns and residents under her supervision. One of the residents gave us the news. I could not go home. I needed more blood in anticipation of the chemotherapy that I was scheduled to receive on Monday. Because I was a "reactor," from now on I would get only washed blood; the blood would be washed, passed through a warmer, and then dripped into my body very slowly. It was too late for all of this today. I would be given the transfusion tomorrow, stay another night in case of a delayed reaction, and if all went well, I could go home on Sunday morning.

My original doctor stepped in to tell us that my bone scan was negative. Was it only yesterday that I had a bone scan? Why wasn't I happy that there was no cancer in my bones? Somehow it didn't seem to matter. This "good news" was cancelled out by my "rare and aggressive" tumor. Suddenly, nothing mattered. It didn't even matter that I wasn't going home today.

I didn't cry. There were no tears left. I had cried enough.

* * *

An exhausted Ralph went home to the children. They presented him with a list of telephone messages. His mother had called. Shayndee and Phyllis had been calling all day. Any word they had asked. What's happening? When is she coming home? Can I call her at the hospital? Should I come?

My parents had called too. They were frantic with worry. They had wanted to get on the first plane as soon as they heard, but Ralph had convinced them not to come. What could they do while I was in the hospital? Better to wait until I would come home so they could be with me and help. Now they were calling to see if I was home yet. They had been sitting next to their telephone all day, waiting to hear my voice from home. Poor Ralph. How would he tell them?

The children had shopped, cooked, and cleaned in anticipation of my coming home. Now they felt cheated. Ralph tried to emphasize the fact that the cancer was confined; it had not spread outside of the uterus. "Rare" and "aggressive" became "unusual," and the chemotherapy was going to be "just to make sure." Nobody was appeased. With Shayndee and Phyllis, he discussed how much to tell my parents. They agreed on what Ralph and I had talked about in the hospital. We would tell them the truth, emphasizing the positive, deemphasizing the negative, and we would try to sound as optimistic and as convincing as possible.

What about the extended family? What about our friends? Do you tell people you have cancer? Do you keep it a secret? We decided not to tell anyone yet. Tomorrow, Ralph and the children would spend the day at the hospital. During the slow-dripping blood transfusion, we would discuss the question, "to tell or not to tell."

My parents, my children, my sisters, called me at the hospital. Everyone maintained control. Everyone, except my mother, who cried unashamedly.

It had been one miserable day.

* * *

Sleep did not come. Whereas last night I had lain awake contemplating my future, tonight I found myself reflecting on the past.

This past year had been difficult for me, both physically and emotionally. My physical problems had begun eleven months ago, in May 1979, when one night I began to hemorrhage during my menstrual period. This had never happened before.

My periods had always been normal, coming every twenty-six to twenty-eight days, lasting from four to six days, with an even, regular flow. This time I was bleeding profusely and passing large purple clots. Ralph called the doctor, I was admitted to the hospital, and a dilation and curettage was performed. The diagnosis: excessive tissue but perfectly normal.

I was told that there was no need for concern. My uterus was cleaned out, everything was in order, and in a month or two I could expect to resume a normal menstrual cycle. I did have one normal period about six weeks after the D & C. Successive periods grew heavier and heavier, they lasted longer and longer, I started passing large clots again. I went back to the doctor—several times. He told me that my pelvic examinations were fine, my Pap smears were coming back negative, the D&C had shown no abnormalities. Not to worry. By November, I had become anemic and I was put on iron supplements.

I had been using the same gynecologist for fourteen years, from the time we moved to West Orange in 1966. Except for when I was pregnant with Jeffrey, I saw him only once a year, for my annual physical exam. I liked him a lot, and more important, I had confidence in him. But I had felt that I needed another opinion, and I made an appointment with one of his partners. The partner checked my medical records, examined me, and confirmed the first doctor's thoughts—no reason for concern.

The heavy bleeding had continued, and Ralph was worried. He wanted me to see another doctor. But who? A hematologist? Another gynecologist? I didn't want to get involved; I didn't want to run from doctor to doctor. And I was so busy —taking care of my family and the house and finishing up my last semester of college at the same time. I told myself I had no reason to worry. My doctor was one of a team of four, and they were not concerned. My pelvic examinations continued to show nothing abnormal. My Pap smears were coming back negative. My recent D&C showed perfectly normal tissue. It was stress, I told myself. Some people get ulcers, some get migraine headaches, some get lower back pain, and some get menstrual irregularities. I knew that stress could play havoc with the body.

And the stress had been mounting. Ralph had been employed by a specialty chemical company that had a division in California, and he was working on a special assignment there. This required frequent travel to the West Coast. Ralph had been asked to relocate to California as the Technical Director of the company's California-based division. We knew very little about family life in California, so we went there for a week to look into communities, housing, and schools. As a result of that trip, we agreed that a move would be possible. But what about the emotional aspects? What about family ties?

At that time, I still had one year of college to complete. Although the company would have liked us to move that winter, they had agreed to wait until June. That way, I could receive my college diploma, the children could finish out the school year, and we would have enough time to make all the necessary arrangements for a cross-country move.

Ralph liked his job. He liked the people he would be working with in California. Here was an opportunity for growth, for advancement, a challenge to build his division into a successful business. He wanted to go with the job.

The children did not want to move to California. Debra and Rachel were in college in New York. They did not want to change schools, and they did not want to leave their friends. Neither did they want to hold us back. Their solution was for us to move and for them to stay back in their college dormitories, eventually finding apartments and jobs in New York. Rhonda was in her sophomore year of high school. There were no dormitories for high school students—Rhonda was stuck with us and very unhappy about changing schools and being taken away from her friends.

Jeffrey was comfortable where he was; there was no way
we could convince him that he could be just as happy in
California as he was in New Jersey.

I was in a quandry. I didn't want to be one of those
women whose husband didn't get ahead because his wife
had held him back. I didn't want to leave Debra and Rachel.
True, they were grown, self-sufficient and able to take
care of themselves, but I still didn't want to move so far
away. We got along well, we talked and confided in each
other, they liked to come home for weekends—how could I
leave them without a home to come back to? And what about
Rhonda? She was happy in school, she had a nice group of
friends, and she was convinced that she would be miserable
in California.

"What do you want?" the girls would often ask me.

I didn't know what I wanted. I wanted to move with my
husband, and I wanted to stay home with my children.

Other considerations included my parents, my sisters and
their families, Ralph's mother and his sister and brothers.
Our parents were getting older. Suppose they got sick?
We would be so far away. Our nieces and nephews were
growing up. When would we see them? I would miss
Shayndee and Phyllis. Long distance phone calls could never
replace our lengthy telephone chats, our shared lunches, our
Saturday night get-togethers. I was happy in West Orange.
We had a nice home, and we had good friends. I didn't want
to move to California where we knew nobody. But what
about Ralph? There was no answer—yet a decision had to
be made. The stress was constant.

Can stress cause cancer? I didn't think so. Not stress
alone anyway. Maybe stress combined with physical abuse
of the body. And there was a time when I had abused my
body. It began in 1964, right after I gave birth to Rhonda.

At my six week checkup, my doctor had told me about all
the virtues of the birth control pill. It was wonderful, he said.
No fuss, no muss. Sex would be spontaneous and my periods

would be predictable. The pill would be convenient, inexpensive, and foolproof, and he wanted me to take it.

I had hesitations. Somehow it didn't seem right, taking a pill every day. I didn't believe in popping pills, especially if there was no illness. But the doctor was so sure it was the best thing for me. There would be no side effects. It was thoroughly tested, and now that it was approved by the FDA, everyone was taking it. It was the thing to do. He was sure I would like it better than any other form of contraception, and he wanted me to try it.

I did. This was in 1964 when the estrogen levels in the pill were very high. It was before it was known that half the dosage was just as effective in preventing conception. It was before anything had been written about the possible side effects. Later, when articles appeared about the safety of the pill and I began to ask questions, I was told not to believe everything I read; I was told that those articles weren't even written by physicians.

I continued to take the birth control pill after we moved to West Orange and I changed doctors. Though I felt no ill effects physically, I was doubting the long term safety of the pill. I discussed my concerns with my new doctor, and we agreed that if I wasn't comfortable with it, I should stop taking it. There were other methods of contraception; the pill wasn't for everyone. I discontinued the pill. I had taken it for two-and-a-half years.

Ten years later, in 1976, when Debra began college and Jeffrey started first grade, I enrolled as a part-time student in Montclair State College. I took classes in what interested me most at the time—health and psychology. In my health class, I did a major project on the birth control pill. My research unveiled a long list of side effects, many of which were unknown to the public. These side effects included weight gain, breast tenderness, nausea, headaches, skin blotchiness, and vaginal discharge. There were also more serious effects, such as complete loss of menstruation, fibroid tumors, diabetes, liver disease, blood clots . . . and cancer. Female cancers, I learned, very often manifest themselves fifteen to twenty years after the initial dose of the pill had been taken.

Two days ago, April 16, 1980, I was diagnosed as having uterine cancer. It was one month before I was to graduate from college. It was the time I would have to make a definite decision on whether or not to move to California. It was sixteen years after I began taking the birth control pill.

Did these things contribute to my developing cancer? Would I ever know? Would anyone?

* * *

I became aware of my wet nightgown. My face, my body, felt hot. I was drenched with sweat. I rang for a nurse.

"I'm soaked," I said when she arrived. "I'm all wet."

The nurse produced a thermometer. It burned in my mouth.

"How high?" I asked when she removed it.

"Very high," she said, and she left to summon another nurse. The second nurse took my temperature again.

"It's a reaction," she announced.

"From what?" I mumbled.

"From the blood transfusion," she informed me.

"I already had a reaction," I told her. "This afternoon I had a rash with welts."

"I know," she said. "That was an immediate reaction. This is a delayed reaction."

I was sponged down, and given medication. My nightgown and my sheets were changed. Ten minutes later I was drenched again and burning up. Another sponge bath, another change of bedclothes. Then chills. I was shivering and trembling. My teeth were chattering. My body was burning. More blankets came, cool compresses were put on my forehead. Still I trembled. My mind wandered; I was disoriented, hallucinating, drifting in and out of reality. A nurse stayed at my side, sponging me down, monitoring my vital signs, and periodically changing my bedclothes. Hot and cold, wet and dry, awareness and nonawareness—this went on until the early hours of the morning, when my temperature finally stabilized.

The immediate crisis was under control, the long-term problem was not. I would not die from the fever; I would have to deal with the cancer.

* * *

Saturday morning brought Ralph and the children to the hospital. In the early afternoon my second blood transfusion was started. The washed, warmed blood was dripped into my body very slowly over a period of about four hours. We watched for a reaction. There was none.

We talked about many things and we made some decisions. As soon as I was strong enough, I would buy a wig. The girls would take me and help me select one. Next week Ralph would go to work late so that he could bring me to the hospital for chemotherapy in the mornings. After the week of chemotherapy was completed, I would go back to school.

Ralph had discussed my finishing school with the doctors yesterday. They had thought that this would not be a good idea. My blood levels would be depressed from the chemo-therapy, and it could be dangerous if I would catch a cold or an infection. Better if I stayed away from crowds and large groups of people, especially young students. I had burst into tears.

"If I'm going to die," I cried, "I want to be buried with my diploma."

Finishing school was very important to me. I had waited a long time to go to college and I had studied diligently for the past four years. A college diploma was the attainment of a long sought-after goal. The doctors reconsidered their decision.

"She's otherwise healthy," one of the partners said to Ralph. "Let her try to lead as normal a life as possible."

By Saturday evening, the next four months of my life had been arranged. In May, I would finish school; in June, I would receive radiation treatments; in July, I would have a radium implant; and in August, I would have surgery. We would not advertise my condition, but neither would we keep it a secret. We would tell our families and our close friends. We would be optimistic, we would think positively, and we would assume that I would have cancer for only four months —until it would be removed with surgery.

On Sunday morning I was finally released. A nurse wheeled me outside of the hospital where we waited for Ralph to come with the car. It was a beautiful day. The sky was so blue, the clouds were so white, the sun was so brilliant. I was happy. I was going home.

* * *

Chapter 2

A WHITE-CLAD NURSE showed us into the office. It was April 21, and we had come to the hospital at nine o'clock for my first chemotherapy treatment. We waited a long time for the oncologist to arrive. I thought about the tigers on the office walls. Why did she choose to decorate her office with pictures of tigers? Do tigers get cancer? Do they get chemotherapy? Do they lose their hair?

Behind the office were two examining rooms.

"Right or left?" the young resident asked me when he arrived with the doctor.

"It doesn't matter," I answered. I was nervous, and my voice quivered. "Can my husband come in with us?"

The answer was yes, and the four of us went into the room on the left. I sat on the examining table, feet dangling, and watched the doctor mix and shake up the chemotherapy solution. She would inject the drug today, she told us. The resident would administer the next four treatments.

My right arm was swabbed, and I looked the other way as the needle was inserted. I felt the cool liquid travel up my arm. I had expected to feel nauseous; instead I felt dizzy.

"I think I'm going to faint," I mumbled.

"Lie back," said a distant voice.

From behind me, strong hands grabbed my shoulders and lowered me down on the examining table. I closed my eyes until the dizziness passed.

"Don't get up until you feel steady," the resident said when I opened my eyes. "You can stay here and rest as long as you want."

"I'm all right now," I said after a few minutes. "I'll try to do better tomorrow."

"Tomorrow you can lie down from the beginning," he said. "I think that will be more comfortable for you."

We all agreed, and the procedure was repeated for the next four days.

All week I felt tired and slightly nauseous. Each day Ralph prepared some lunch for me before he left for work, but I usually couldn't eat it. I found that if I napped in the afternoon, I could muster up enough energy to prepare dinner for the family, but right after dinner, I was overwhelmingly tired again. I needed a lot of sleep and just a bare minimum of bland, dry food. I never did get violently ill. I was grateful for that, and by the end of the week I decided that chemotherapy wasn't all that horrible.

* * *

I stepped out of the shower. I took two large bath towels off the rack, and I wrapped my body in one and my wet hair in the other. When I was dry, I put on my nightgown and stood in front of the mirror, waiting for the mist to clear. I unwrapped the towel from around my head.

I stared at myself in disbelief.

My hair had matted together in tangled clumps all over my head. There were places where I could see my scalp showing through my hair.

"Ralph!" I screamed.

It was Saturday night, and we had planned a quiet evening at home. Debra was away for the weekend, Rachel was getting ready for a date, and Ralph was watching television with Rhonda and Jeffrey while I showered. Now he came bounding up the stairs.

"Oh my God," he exclaimed. "What a mess!"

I started to cry.

"Don't get uspet," he said sympathetically. "We can fix it."

He took my brush and started to work on one of the clumps. It didn't unravel. He tried a comb. It didn't work.

"That's a rough one," he said. "Don't worry. We'll try another one."

The more he tried to unravel, the more hair fell out. Tears trickled down my face.

"I'll call Rachel," Ralph said. "She knows all about hair. She'll know what to do."

Rachel had beautiful hair. Golden brown, straight, and falling almost to the waist, with a smattering of bangs on her forehead. Rachel's hair glowed. We called it her crowning glory.

Now she came into my room with an assortment of brushes. She worked on me for half an hour while Ralph looked on and I whimpered. It was to no avail. I still had matted clumps. The brushes were full of hair, and there was hair all over the floor.

"We'll have to cut it," Ralph said.

"No!" I cried back.

"What's our choice?" he said. "You can't go around like that."

Rachel went for the scissors.

"Not too much, Rach," I pleaded. "Maybe if you just make a few snips by the knots, the rest will unravel."

Rachel lifted a clump of matted hair. The entire clump came off in her hand. We watched with amazement, the tears streaming down my face. Rachel kept trying. Clump after tangled clump separated from my head and fell around me on the bathroom floor.

I looked back in the mirror. My head was checkered with patches of sparse black hair and pale bald spots. I looked awful.

By Monday, almost all of my hair had fallen out. I was

embarrassed for anyone to see me. I would have to start wearing my wig.

* * *

I hated the wig. It was beautiful, it looked good on me, and no one who didn't know could tell it was a wig. Still I hated it. It felt unnatural to go around with phony hair on my head. I felt as if I was trying to fool people, to make them think that I still had beautiful black shoulder-length hair.

I bought some scarves. The scarves became my daily headcovering, and the wig was relegated to special occasions. Only when I went someplace where it would have been totally inappropriate to wear a scarf, did I resort to wearing the wig.

Bald, scarved, or wigged—every glance in a mirror reminded me that I had cancer.

* * *

The next step was a "planning" meeting with the radiotherapy department. My course of radiation would be planned, and I would begin the treatments two days later.

My medical history was reviewed, and I was examined and X-rayed. The X-rays were illuminated on a wall board, and using them as a guide, the radiotherapist measured me. All kinds of gadgets were placed on my abdomen as I lay on the examining table. With what looked like a Magic Marker, purple lines were drawn on my body from below the chest area to the upper legs. Numbers, x's, and various other signs and symbols completed the decoration. My body looked like an assortment of tic-tac-toe games. I was asked to turn over, and a similar procedure was done on my back and buttocks. Now the technicians would know exactly where to radiate.

The X-ray machine to be used would be the linear accelerator, which would give a maximum dose of megavoltage radiation beneath the skin rather than on it. Radiation would enter my body from four different angles. Every other day I would lie on my back and the X-rays would be beamed from both the left and the right sides. On the alternating days, I would lie on my stomach and the procedure would be repeated. The beams would meet each other where the tumor was located. Changing the direction of the incoming beams would allow the tumor to get sufficient radiation yet would keep destruction of normal tissue to a minimum.

I would be given two hundred rads a day for twenty days—a total of four thousand rads of radiation. This would take four weeks, since the radiotherapy department operated only five days a week, Monday through Friday. Twice each week I would go to the blood lab for a CBC, a complete blood count. This would be necessary because the radiation depresses the blood levels. If the blood cells would drop below a certain point, the treatments would have to be interrupted. Though most patients on radiation require only a weekly CBC, I would have to be checked twice a week since I was taking oral chemotherapy, which also depresses blood levels, at the same time that I was being given the radiation.

My treatments would begin in two days, on May 7.

"What about the long-term side effects of so much radiation?" I asked the radiotherapist. "Couldn't the treatments alone cause another cancer twenty years from now?"

"Yes," he answered honestly. "But we can't worry about that now. We can't deny you treatments for an existing tumor because of the possibility of side effects in twenty years. We have to destroy the tumor you have now."

I had to agree. If I wanted to live another twenty years, I thought, then I have no choice but to submit to these treatments.

Before leaving, we met with the head radiation nurse, and

we arranged for my treatments to be given early in the morning. That way, Ralph could take me before he went to work. I was told not to wash off the ink marks on my body. They had to stay on during the whole course of treatment since they showed the technician where to aim the radiation.

I noticed the poster on the waiting room wall. It was a picture of Snoopy holding up a big towel on which was written in bold, colorful letters, "DON'T WASH OFF YOUR MARKS!"

* * *

Chairs were lined up against the walls in the waiting room. Interspersed between the chairs were square tables on which magazines were arranged. In one corner was a low round table with little chairs for children. Picture books, coloring books, crayons, and puzzles lay haphazardly on the table. In another corner was the nurse's desk, and at the front of the desk was a yellow pad with two columns. Each patient signed in under one of the two headings: "To see the Doctor" or "For Treatment."

I added my name to the list in the "For Treatment" column and sat down. People all around were either chatting quietly or reading magazines. No one wore a scarf.

"Why am I the only one with no hair?" I whispered to Ralph.

"You're not," he whispered back. "Some people are wearing wigs."

I looked around. There were men, women, and children of all ages. Everyone looked perfectly normal.

"Do you think all these people have cancer?" I asked Ralph.

"No," he replied. "Some people are probably here with relatives."

"I hope so," I said. "I hope we don't have to wait for all these people to have treatments."

I picked up a magazine and tried to read. I couldn't concentrate, so I just held the magazine on my lap and worried about what would happen when I went inside.

"Elaine Nussbaum," called a nurse's voice.

I got up, but Ralph didn't.

"Come on," I said, pulling his hand.

"I can't go in there," he said. "I'll wait out here for you."

"Come with me," I begged, starting to feel panicky. "I'm sure you can come in to the next room. Try."

I tugged at his hand, and he got up. We were ushered into the next waiting room.

It was a long corridor-like room that ended in a large rectangular shape. On one wall were machines with blinking lights and clicking sounds. On the two other walls were giant-sized doors which opened into the treatment rooms. On one door was a sign that read, "Cobalt," on the other door a sign read, "Linear Accelerator." A light above each door glowed red or green.

We sat down in the row of chairs in the corridor. On the wall opposite us was a display of posters, all bearing the same message, "DON'T WASH OFF YOUR MARKS!" Here the patients weren't reading or chatting; they just sat, waiting. A woman next to me was wearing a paper gown instead of a blouse, and through the arm holes I could see the purple marks around her breast area. A man had his tic-tac-toe designs on one side of his face and head, and another man had his on his neck and upper chest. Breast cancer? Brain tumor? Throat or thyroid cancer? I was grateful that my marks were covered with clothing.

The head radiation nurse came over to me. My heart started to pound. It wasn't my turn yet; there were still some people ahead of me.

"This is your first treatment," she said kindly.

I nodded.

"Come with me," she said.

I followed her down the corridor to where a scale stood. I hadn't noticed the scale when we came in.

"Would you like to take your shoes off?" she asked me.

"Should I?"

"If you want to. Or you can leave them on. It's up to you."

I took off my shoes and stepped on the scale.

The nurse opened her folder and wrote down my weight. I saw my picture on the inside cover of the folder. Did someone take my picture at the planning session? I didn't remember.

"Why do you have to weigh me?" I asked the nurse.

She explained that it was important for me to maintain my normal weight. Maintaining my weight would indicate that I was getting enough calories each day. Protein and calorie needs are greater during illness and treatment than they usually are, she explained, and it was important that I eat a high protein, high calorie, diet. It was also important that I get enough rest, she continued. Most people can go ahead with their normal activities during radiation, but some patients find that they tire very easily and need a lot of rest. Fatigue is a very common side effect of radiation. Any side effects that I might experience, she said, should be brought to her attention, and I would be advised as to how to deal with them.

"What kind of side effects should I expect?" I asked.

Most patients experience no serious difficulty during treatment, she told me, and if problems do appear, they usually develop after a period of time. They may include fatigue, nausea, vomiting, diarrhea, dizziness, and skin irritation. It was very important, she said, to protect the treatment area. I should not wash with soap or put on salves, powders, bandages, or medications. I should not apply hot or cold objects, I should not rub, scrub, or scratch, and I should not expose the area to the sun. Most important, I should not wash off the ink marks used to indicate the target.

"What about a shower?" I asked. "I can't go a whole month without taking a shower."

If I wanted to shower, she told me, I should wrap some

plastic around the treatment area to protect it. I should use lukewarm water, and if the area would get a little wet, I should gently pat it dry. I should also remember not to wear tight-fitting or irritating clothing over the treated area. I should not worry if my skin turns a shade darker than its normal color as this is usually a temporary condition.

She assured me that radiation is invisible and painless. The machine would point the radiation at the part of my body to be treated, and I would not feel anything at all.

I returned to my chair to await my turn. In a few minutes, the light over the "Linear Accelerator" door blinked green, and two technicians came to escort me into the treatment room.

* * *

The gigantic machine shone in the dimly lit room. We walked over to the cot that was near the machine, and I was told to lie down on my back. The cot was then wheeled under the machine's lighted cylinder.

I did not have to undress. I was asked to lower my slacks to my pelvis and to raise my blouse to my chest. The technicians then checked my marks, did some measuring on my abdomen, and drew some more lines. Then they stepped back, and I watched as one of them picked up a Polaroid camera and snapped a picture of my exposed area.

"For your folder," he said as we waited to see if the picture would be acceptable.

Apparently it was. They then checked my position on the cot and did some more measuring. The X-ray equipment was adjusted, the machine was focused, and the controls were set. I was told to lie very still—not to move at all. I could just relax and breathe normally. The treatment would take only a few minutes. They left the room, and the giant door closed behind them.

The machine clicked on, and a slight whirring sound began. Lights blinked on and off on what looked like an instrument panel against the wall. I closed my eyes and thought about the two hundred rads of radiation bombarding my body. Silent destruction. Killing the good along with the bad, I thought. I was scared. Suppose the machine didn't shut itself off?

The whirring sound suddenly stopped. Silence. It broke, I thought in panic. The machine broke. Why doesn't someone come in and rescue me? I lay still, afraid to move. I was stiff with apprehension.

A click, and the cylinder that was pointing at the right side of my body began to move. Outward it went, then upward, and crossing over my body it positioned itself on my left side, pointing inward. Another click, and the whirring sound began again.

It took only a few minutes, but it seemed like hours. Finally the machine shut off, the door was pushed open, and the technicians came in to get me. Unknown to me then, they had watched me during the entire treatment time on a closed circuit television system just outside the treatment room. They had not abandoned me.

People were lined up in the corridor, waiting their turns. Does this go on all day, I wondered. Do these two machines run all day long, five days a week, all through the year? This is just one hospital in New Jersey. What about all the other hospitals across the country? Do they all have cobalt machines and linear accelerators? Do they all have people lined up all the time, awaiting a turn? Do so many people have cancer?

A patient was being wheeled in on a stretcher, with all the intravenous apparatus attached. A nurse and two attendants accompanied him. That's why the doors are so big, I thought. They have to accommodate wheelchairs and stretchers.

Before I left, I was given a green spiral-bound book of eating hints. It contained recipes and tips for better nutrition during cancer treatment. Included in the book were recipes that were high in nutritional value, easy to prepare, and abundant in protein and calories. These would help me in my attempt to maintain my weight.

What would be so terrible if I lost a few pounds? I wondered. I was always trying to lose a few pounds. So were Debra, Rachel, and Rhonda. So were Shayndee and Phyllis. So were most of my friends. Wasn't everyone?

Rhonda and I had been weighing in together every week.

"How much, Rhon?" I always asked when she stepped off the scale.

Rhonda always weighed five or six pounds less than I did. She had a perfect figure; whatever she put on looked beautiful on her. So what if I had a figure like Rhonda? I would go down a size. We could share our skirts. Losing weight, I thought, would be the least of my problems. It might even be a benefit.

Once every week I would be weighed. Once every week I would see a doctor. Twice each week, Tuesdays and Fridays, I would have blood drawn. I would remember not to wash off my marks. I would do exactly as I was told.

One treatment was finished. I had nineteen more to look forward to.

* * *

I would have to rearrange my schedule at school. This was my last college semester, and I was student-teaching at the local high school. I had become a Business Education major, leaving my health and psychology interests behind. "What will you do with a degree in health or psychology?" Ralph had asked me when I had accumulated enough credits to declare a major. At that time, I had no intention of continuing my education past the college level. My goal was a college degree, followed by a job.

A degree in the health field meant a Home Economics major which necessitated taking classes in family relations, meal planning, consumer economics, and other home-family-consumer type classes. I had been a housewife for twenty years and I had raised four children. It hadn't made much sense for me to major in Home Economics at that point in my life. I already was a home economist.

I had considered psychology. Certainly, my interest was there, and I knew I would enjoy the courses. But what kind of job could I get with an undergraduate degree in psychology? I would need a master's degree, I thought, and possibly even a doctorate. What would be the point of investing four years in college if I couldn't get a job afterwards? Ralph and I had studied the college catalogue and discussed the pros and cons of the available majors.

We had decided on Business Education. Teaching, we had agreed, would be a perfect job for me. I would be home every day before the children, and on snowy, hazardous-driving days school would be closed. I would be off every school vacation and every summer. I could teach teenagers in a public or private high school, or I could teach adults in a business school. If I found that I didn't enjoy teaching, I could always be an overqualified secretary.

I had become a Business Education major. I had taken courses in secretarial skills such as typewriting, stenography, and office procedures, and I had taken business courses such as business management, business law, marketing, and accounting. Now, in my last semester, I was teaching five classes a day to junior and senior high school students.

My school day began at 7:40 in the morning, and I returned home shortly after 3:00 in the afternoon. Every evening I prepared lesson plans for the next day. These lesson plans had to be perfectly typed. Shopping, cooking, cleaning, laundry, and other family duties were squeezed into any remaining time. And now, I had to reschedule my day around my morning radiation treatments.

The high school staff was very cooperative. I dropped my early morning accounting class and picked up an extra class in teh afternoon. On this new schedule, I didn't have to be in school until 9:30.

Every morning I went to the hospital for radiation. I had about half an hour at home to rest, exchange my scarf for my wig, and drive to school to teach.

I was determined to achieve my goal of holding a college diploma. I would not let the cancer snatch this away from me. Ralph and the children took over the household responsibilities, and I put all my energies into completing my student-teaching.

On May 21, 1980, I graduated from Montclair State College, Summa Cum Laude, with a grade point average of 3.9, the highest average in the Business Education Department.

I had fulfilled a dream. I had achieved a goal. Certainly, this was not the time for me to die of cancer. I had too much to live for. I would set other goals. I would get a job. I would dance at Jeffrey's Bar-Mitzvah. How could I die and leave a little boy who hasn't even reached the age of Bar-Mitzvah? I would not allow that to happen. I would raise my children to adulthood. I would not make my husband a widower, nor would I bring grief to my parents. I would finish my radiation treatments, I would submit to and recover from surgery, and then I would not have cancer anymore. I made my decision. I would not die.

* * *

What happens to a family when Mother can no longer function in her usual role? Who does the shopping, the cleaning, the laundry? Who prepares breakfast and dinner, and who packs lunches for school? Who drives to the library, to the dentist, to little league practice? Who helps with homework? Who is always there to listen, to advise, to share?

The cumulative effects of the radiation and the chemotherapy made me weak and chronically tired. I napped every morning and again in the afternoon, and I returned to my bed immediately after dinner. I was overwhelmed with fatigue. And with guilt. Guilt for falling down on the job. For not being able to take care of my family. For causing such an upheaval in their lives. For causing them so much worry, stress, and fear.

Ralph was running himself ragged, working all day and handling the shopping, cooking, cleaning, laundry, and telephone calls in the evenings. Rhonda tried to relieve him but he wanted to do it all himself. Rhonda felt sorry for him—he was so busy all day and all night. She felt sorry for me. She knew how it hurt me to feel so helpless, to be unable to do the things that I always did so routinely.

Debra and Rachel were both in college and feeling that they should be home. The school semester was coming to an end, papers had to be completed, and final exams had to be studied for. Ralph assured them that they didn't have to keep coming home, that everything was under control. Still, they felt guilty.

Coming home in the evenings created problems too. They felt that by coming home often, they were only making more busy work for Ralph. He would have to pick them up at the bus stop and bring them back late at night or early the next morning. He would have to prepare dinner. It was a catch-22 situation; they felt guilty coming home and they felt guilty being away.

Feelings of guilt were coupled with feelings of fear and uncertainty. We were all trying so hard to believe that our situation was temporary, that after my surgery all would be well and we would resume normal living again. We could think this on an intellectual level, we could try to believe it, we could hope it would be so. But we could not control our deepest fear. What if the cancer had spread?

My illness was consuming everyone's time, energies, and thoughts. Everything else became inconsequential. What difference did it make if supper was a cheese sandwich, if nobody folded the laundry, if a skirt and sweater didn't match, if you missed your bus or got caught in the rain? So what if you botched a final exam, forgot to hand in a paper, or got a "B" instead of an "A" in your favorite subject. Who cared? What difference did it make when your mother might be dying?

One thing was on everyone's mind—what would be revealed at the time of the surgery?

* * *

The radiation shrank the tumor—but not enough. I would need a radium implant, internal radiation, to complete the job.

I didn't want it.

It was necessary, I was told. My oncologist and my team of radiotherapists had decided that I must submit to yet another violation of my body.

On June 24, 1980, one day after my twenty-third wedding anniversary, I was wheeled into the operating room and put under general anesthesia. A hollow applicator was inserted in my body and packed into position with medicated gauze. I was then taken to my room, where the radium was put into the applicator.

I became radioactive. The radioactive material inside me could pass through my body into the surrounding area, so my room, too, contained radiation. A sign was posted on the door, "DANGER, RADIOACTIVE AREA." A tag was placed on my arm, "RADIOACTIVE MATERIAL."

My visitors were limited to Ralph. Ralph was allowed to

come once a day and stay for only ten minutes. He had to stand at least six feet away from my bed in order to minimize his exposure to the radiation. No other visitors were allowed.

Phyllis came anyway. She didn't tell anyone she was coming, she just appeared. She arrived with a shopping bag filled with cake and magazines.

"I hope you're not pregnant, Phyl," I said. "There's a lot of radiation in here."

"I hope I'm not pregnant, too," she answered, "And not just because of the radiation."

She put the shopping bag down by my bed.

"I won't kiss you," she said. And she went to stand in the doorway.

We chatted for ten minutes and then agreed she should leave.

"Thanks for the magazines and the cake," I said. "There's a lot here. Maybe I'll send some cake home with Ralph for the kids."

"That's what I had in mind," said Phyllis. "There'll be one less thing Ralph will have to buy for the weekend."

Suddenly the same thought occurred to both of us. Could the children, or anyone else, eat the cake after it had been in the radioactive room? Was there radiation in the cake? Was it safe to eat?

"I'll ask a nurse," said Phyllis.

"Wait a minute," I called. "You're not supposed to be here."

We didn't know what to do with the cake. We decided not to take any chances. We wouldn't give it to the children. We wouldn't give it to anyone. Phyllis disposed of the cake, and we never told anyone what happened.

The children really wanted to visit me, despite the rules. Ralph and I decided that they absolutely should not come. We didn't want them to be exposed to any radiation at all. We had enough problems. Jeffrey wanted to know if he could at least give Ralph some of his batteries to take to the hospital. He thought he could have them recharged on my radioactive body.

Intra-uterine implants are usually left in place anywhere from twelve to seventy-two hours. Mine was a seventy-two hour ordeal. During this time, I lay perfectly flat on my back. I could turn my head from side to side, I could raise my arms, and I could wiggle my toes. Nothing more. Everything from my neck to my ankles remained motionless. A catheter was inserted to drain my urine, and I was given medication to stop bowel function. I was put on a special diet of bland, fiberless food and lots of liquid. In other words, mush.

My hospital care was quite different than usual. The nurses came into my room with Geiger counters and never stayed more than a few minutes. My sheets were not changed and I was not bathed. My room was entered to deliver my food and medication, to empty my urine bag, and to take my temperature with a disposable thermometer. Nobody stayed to chat.

My first attempt at eating was a disaster. The tray was placed on a table by my bed where, supposedly, I would be able to reach the food without moving my body. I reached for the paper cup of apple juice. I lifted my head and tried to bring the cup to my lips. The juice spilled all over my face. I picked up my plastic fork and stuck it into some mush in a little plastic container. The mush fell off the fork and onto my bed. There was another container on the tray. I couldn't open it. I rang for a nurse.

"I can't eat," I said when she appeared in the doorway. "I lose it before it gets to my mouth."

"I'll call someone to help you," she said.

A young nurse's aid came in. A device to measure the level of radiation in the room was strapped to her pocket. She kept checking to make sure it was there. She looked scared.

"What do you need help with?" she asked me.

"Something to drink," I answered.

She picked up my paper cup of apple juice, now half empty, and held it to my face. It ran down my chin.

"Turn your head to the side," she said.

We tried again. The juice trickled down the side of my mouth.

"Let's try some food," she suggested.

She put a blob of food on the fork and brought it to my mouth. I swallowed with a gulp. It tasted awful, whatever it was. She refilled the fork. And then her Geiger counter went off. She dropped the forkful of food on the tray and ran out of the room. She never came back.

When Ralph came for his ten-minute visit, the uneaten food was still there. Ralph spoke to the head nurse and demanded that someone help me with breakfast and lunch. He offered to do dinner. He purchased a box of bendable straws which enabled me to sip if someone held the cup in the proper position. He also brought me some decent food. It was plain and low in fiber, but at least it tasted like food. All day I looked forward to Ralph's ten-minute visit in the evening.

My sanity was preserved by the presence of my roommate, Hattie. Hattie and I were both having seventy-two hour implants, and we were being treated by the same radiotherapist. Although implant patients are usually kept in private rooms, our doctor scheduled our insertions back to back so that we would have each other's company. Both of us were surprised when we woke up from the anesthesia and found a roommate in the next bed.

Hattie was twenty years my senior and twice my size. She had a sunny disposition, a good sense of humor, and she never complained. We quickly became good friends.

You can do a lot of talking in seventy-two hours, and Hattie and I did. We talked about our cancers, our treatments, our doctors, our families and their reactions, and our own hopes and fears. We talked about the hospital routine, and about how we felt lying there for seventy-two hours with nothing to do but look at the urine bags filling up at the side of our beds. We hardly slept. When one of us stirred in the night, the other was always awake to ask, "Are you all right?" When one of us felt uncomfortable, the other always offered to ring for a nurse. When one of us felt sad or depressed, the other would listen, would sympathize, would understand.

The implants were removed right in our room. We were given medication for pain, and about half an hour later the doctor came in to remove the applicator and the packing. The curtain between our beds was drawn, and Hattie's implant was removed first.

"It doesn't hurt much," she called from her side of the curtain.

Either she was being kind or her pain tolerance was better than mine. It hurt plenty.

When the curtain was pulled back, Hattie was sitting up in her bed. She rested a few minutes, then got off the bed, walked alone to the bathroom, and emerged a few minutes later washed, dressed, and wearing make-up.

I tried to sit up and I felt dizzy. I waited a few minutes and tried again. I couldn't get up. Hattie rang for a nurse. I was helped to a sitting position and told to just sit and dangle my legs for a few minutes. The dizziness passed. The nurse helped me off the bed. My legs buckled and I almost toppled over. I couldn't stand. I was put back to bed.

The nurse left and returned a short while later with another nurse. They both helped me to a sitting position, then to a standing position, and slowly they walked me around the room a few times. They left me standing by the bed and told me to practice walking around it while holding on until I could let go and walk on my own.

Hattie took my arm and walked me over to the bathroom.

"Hattie," I called from behind the closed door. "Please don't go away. I don't feel too steady in here."

I leaned against the sink and looked in the mirror. My face looked pale, my eyes were sunken and cloudy, my scarf was twisted in a hotchpotch around my bald head. I had not washed my hands and face or brushed my teeth in three days. I looked like I had felt for these past seventy-two hours—dehumanized.

I washed myself, making a mess in the bathroom. When I finished, Hattie took my arm again and I hobbled back to the bed.

"I'll help you get dressed," Hattie offered.

"I'm too exhausted," I said. "I think I'll just lie here and wait for Ralph."

Hattie's husband arrived, and before we said good-bye, we exchanged telephone numbers and promised to stay in touch. And we did. From June to November, we spoke to each other on the phone two or three times every week.

Ralph took me home, and I spent the next few days trying to regain some strength. I was tired, weak, and mentally cloudy. I was told to eat well, get plenty of rest, and to try to build myself up again. Except for the chemotherapy that I was taking orally, I would have no other treatments until surgery.

My surgery was scheduled for August 5.

* * *

The tension was building. The knot in my stomach and the fear in my heart grew heavier with each passing day. I was scared of the surgery. I found myself imagining all kinds of catastrophies. The knife would slip. My heart would stop beating. A blood clot would develop. I wouldn't be revived from the anesthesia. Dying on the operating table seemed a real possibility. Should I say good-bye to my children, I

wondered. Should I tell them how much I love them? Should I
tell them to try to remember me as I used to be—a happy
and loving mother?

Debra and Rachel would be home for the summer. Since
beginning college, they had held various part-time jobs during the school year and full-time jobs during the summers.
Now Debra took a summer job in a jewelry store, and Rachel
would work in a pencil factory. They would live at home and
we would face this summer together.

Rhonda had planned to go to overnight camp as a waitress,
but now she was changing her mind. She thought it might be
better to try to get a job near home and spend the summer
with the family.

What kind of job could you get, Rhon?" I asked her.
"You're only fifteen and you don't drive yet."

I knew she felt guilty about leaving. And I felt guilty
keeping her back. I had already placed a tremendous burden
on my young daughter. I wanted her at least to have a nice
summer.

"All your friends will be away at camp," I told Rhonda.
"Go and have a good time. It will make me happy."

I promised that we would speak on the phone regularly
and that we would all come up to camp on visiting day, a
week and a half before my surgery, and spend the day
together. Rhonda agreed to go to camp.

Ralph and I were in disagreement about Jeffrey. Last
summer he had gone to day camp at our local YMHA, and
he was registered to go again. Ralph wanted to send him to
overnight camp. It wouldn't be good for me, Ralph thought,
to have to worry about where Jeffrey would stay when I was
in the hospital and about who would take care of him while
I was recuperating. In camp he would be taken care of; we
wouldn't have to worry about him and he wouldn't have to
worry about me.

But I would worry. Jeffrey was ten years old, too young,
I thought, to go away for eight weeks. What bothered me

even more than sending him away at such a young age was the reasoning behind it. It wasn't because he wanted to go to overnight camp. It wasn't because I thought he would have such a good time there. It was because I wouldn't be able to take care of him. This inability was hurting me.

My parents were planning to come up from Florida at the time of the surgery and stay for as long as I needed them. I could take care of Jeffrey in July, I thought, and my Mom could take over in August. Ralph still felt that it would be better for all of us if Jeffrey went to camp.

I consented. Maybe Ralph was right, I rationalized. In camp Jeffrey would be busy all day, and he would not have to come home to a sick mother every night. He would not see me confined to bed or in pain. Maybe he would forget about cancer and just have a good time. Maybe it really would be better for him to be away at this time. Maybe camp would be a positive experience for him. Some of his friends were going and he thought he would have a good time if he went too. We registered Jeffrey in overnight camp.

I read twelve books in July—all about cancer. In between my naps I would sit outside and read. I read about all kinds of cancer, not only uterine, and I became familiar with the many theories of cancer development, control, and cure. The treatments I was undergoing were somewhat standard, I learned; chemotherapy, radiation, and surgery were the only weapons medical science had to fight this dread disease. Some people survived and some didn't. I tried to be optimistic.

It was nice to have Debra and Rachel home, and with their schedules somewhat relaxed for the summer, Shayndee and Phyllis were able to come visit me often. Shayndee was a nursery school teacher, and she spent a good part of her summer vacation with me. Shayndee did not dwell on the cancer or the upcoming surgery. We talked about lighter things, and with her wit and her keen sense of humor, she managed to cheer me up a little. Shayndee's visits brightened my days.

Phyllis was a psychologist. Phyllis felt that it was important to talk about it—to let the feelings come out. Phyllis and I spent a lot of time talking about my emotions: anger, guilt, fear, self-pity. Phyllis assured me that these were all okay.

I had stopped going to Synagogue on Saturdays, partially because it was a long walk and I was too tired, and partially because I was losing my faith. How could I praise and exalt God when He was doing this to me? I had cancer, I might die, I was suffering, my family was suffering; for what should I thank God? But as the impending surgery came closer, I was getting more and more frightened. I was afraid to alienate God. Maybe if I don't desert Him, I thought, He won't desert me. I tried to pray, but I found it difficult to concentrate. I would go to Synagogue, I decided. On the Saturday before the surgery, I would go and I would try to regain some faith. I would pray hard, I would beg for my life, and maybe God would listen and help me.

I overslept. By the time I arrived at the Synagogue, the service was over. I felt defeated. I hadn't prayed with the congregation. I hadn't begged God for mercy. I had missed my last chance. I went straight to the ladies room and cried.

My friend Florence came in and found me bawling.

"Don't cry, Elaine," she said, putting her arm around me. "Everything's going to be all right."

"I missed it," I sobbed. "I came too late and I missed the whole thing."

"You can pray at home," Florence said. "God hears you wherever you are. Try not to cry."

I buried my face in her shoulder and cried harder.

"Want my sunglasses?" Florence asked, producing a pair.

"No thanks," I answered, trying to regain my composure. "I'll be all right. Thanks for being here."

"Ralph got nervous when he couldn't find you," she said. "He sent me to look for you."

Ralph was waiting right outside the ladies room.

"I missed it," I told him somberly. "I came too late. I didn't pray a single word."

"It's okay," he assured me. "I prayed enough for both of us."

Ralph took my hand, and we walked home together in silence.

On Monday, August 4, I checked into the hospital. Early the next morning my doctor would perform a total abdominal hysterectomy and a bilateral salpingo-oophorectomy, the removal of my uterus, ovaries, and fallopian tubes. Ralph, Debra, and Rachel would wait in the hospital. The others would wait by their phones.

The time had come. Tomorrow we would know. I was ready.

* * *

Chapter 3

T HE ANESTHESIOLOGIST STALKED INTO MY ROOM.
"Elaine Nussbaum?" he asked.
I nodded.

"I'll be giving you anesthesia tomorrow morning," he said, and I'd like to ask you some questions now."

"Okay," I said.

He flipped through my chart and a frown crossed his face.

"When was the last time you had blood drawn?" he asked.

"This afternoon," I told him. "Shortly after I was admitted."

"Your blood levels are very low," he said. "I'm not sure we can put you under tomorrow."

My stomach knotted, a lump rose in my chest, and my legs turned to water.

"Why not?" I blurted out.

"When was the last time you had chemotherapy?" he asked me. He was looking at my records on his clipboard.

"In April," I said. "I had five treatments of Cytoxan, intravenously."

"And your radiation was from May 7 to June 4?" he queried.

"That's right," I said. "And I also had a seventy-two hour radium implant, June 24 to 27."

"Hmm," he murmured. "That wouldn't account for this blood picture."

"Are you taking any medication now?" he asked.

"No," I answered. "Just vitamins and the oral chemotherapy."

"Oral chemotherapy?" he exclaimed, shifting his eyes from

the clipboard to me. "When was the last time you took oral chemotherapy?"

"This afternoon," I answered. "I take Cytoxan three times a day. One hundred fifty milligrams, fifty at each meal."

"Well that explains these low blood levels," he said.

"Are they too low to operate?" I asked in a shaky voice.

"They might be," he said. "Usually we stop chemotherapy a while before surgery so that blood levels can return to an acceptable level. But I'll talk it over with your doctor."

He got up to leave.

"Wait!" I called after him, trying to control the panic I was feeling. "When will you know? Will someone come tell me tonight?"

"Someone will tell you," he said.

"Please," I pleaded. "Please let me know tonight. Please let me know in either case."

"We'll let you know," he promised. "Now I'm going to try to locate your doctor and find out why you've been taking chemotherapy up until surgery."

I wanted the surgery tomorrow. I wanted it to be done with—over. I couldn't bear to go through this again: the expectation, the mounting tension, the frazzled nerves that accompanied the final days. I didn't want a reprieve. I wanted the surgery now.

My roommate was telling me that surgery wasn't so wonderful. A lung cancer patient, she had had surgery more than a month ago, and she was still in the hospital. She had had radiation in another hospital prior to her surgery, and the radiation had burned her esophagus resulting in an inability to eat. Now she was being fed intravenously, and every few hours she was brought a calorie-rich chocolate milk shake which she was supposed to drink but didn't. She wanted to go home, but the hospital wouldn't release her until she could eat on her own.

I found it hard to look at her. She was pale and gaunt, her eyes were sunken and lifeless, and a small amount of sparse blond hair jutted up on her head. She looked like she was near death and she sounded as sick as she looked; her labored speech was punctuated with gags and coughs. She tried to make conversation, but I was too wrapped up in my own problems to be friendly. I wanted the cancer out—now. I wanted to get out of this hospital. I didn't want to end up like my roommate.

A handsome young man walked into my room.

"Elaine Nussbaum?" he asked.

"That's me," I answered.

"I'm a senior resident in gynecological oncology," he said. "I'll be assisting in your surgery tomorrow, and I want to tell you what the procedure. . . ."

"Surgery tomorrow!" I interrupted him. "Will I have the surgery tomorrow?"

"Isn't that what you're here for?" he asked me.

"Yes," I answered, and I told him about my visit from the anesthesiologist.

He nodded in acknowledgment. He told me that my oncologist, radiotherapist, anesthesiologist, and the head of pathology were discussing my case right now. He was pretty certain that the decision would be to operate. We talked for a while about the procedure, and when he left I felt better and reassured.

Ralph came and I told him what had happened. Together we waited for more news.

The anesthesiologist returned with his clipboard.

"We're all set for tomorrow morning," he said.

"Is it dangerous?" Ralph asked him. "I don't want you to operate if there's any danger to her. Have you ever anesthesized other patients with such low blood levels?"

"Sometimes we see this with leukemia patients," he answered. "We have to evaluate each situation separately and there are many considerations other than blood levels. In this case, we feel that it's best to go ahead."

"Good." I chimed in. "I'm glad."

The anesthesiologist proceeded to ask me some questions. Had I had anesthesia before? Had I had any ill effects from it? Was I sensitive to any drugs? Did I have any allergies? Do I have any history of liver or kidney disease? Had I taken any tranquilizers, antidepressants, or sedatives lately?

"How do you feel tonight?" was his last question. "Are you nervous?"

"Very," I answered honestly.

"I'll prescribe some Valium for you," he offered. "It will help to relax you and you'll be able to get a good night's sleep."

"No thanks," I answered. "I'm not that nervous."

"Valium's okay, hon," Ralph said. "I take it sometimes when I can't sleep."

"I don't want it," I insisted. "I'm sure I'll be able to sleep without it."

Strange, I thought to myself. I've taken hundreds of milligrams of chemotherapy, I've been bombarded with megadoses of radiation, tomorrow I would be getting deep anesthesia, and I'm refusing a little Valium because I don't believe in taking pills. Very strange, but nevertheless, I didn't want it.

The anesthesiologist got up to leave. He bade me good night and he shook hands with Ralph.

"Take care of her," Ralph pleaded, his voice shaking.

"Don't worry," the anesthesiologist said kindly. "She'll be in the best of hands."

* * *

"You'll have to remove your nail polish," the nurse said.

"Why?" I asked. "It's just clear polish."

"The doctors have to be able to see if your nails turn blue," she said. And she produced a wad of cotton and a bottle of polish remover and began working on my nails.

Another nurse appeared with a needle.

"This will help you relax," she said. "It'll make you drowsy, but it won't put you to sleep."

I got drowsy right after the injection.

"Will you be here?" I asked Ralph, Debra, and Rachel who were standing by the foot of my bed. "Will you be here when I come back?"

Ralph came over and picked up my limp hand.

"We'll be here," he said.

"Please be here," I begged him. My eyes were filling up with tears. "I'll feel safer if I know that you're here."

"I'll be here," he promised, and he planted a kiss on my forehead. . . .

Everything was getting blurry. A cap was placed on my head, and then I was moving. My bed was wheeled into the corridor, then into the elevator, and down. Another corridor, and then through the swinging doors that read, "OPERAT-ING ROOMS. NO ADMITTANCE." I was parked next to the wall.

Nurses in green uniforms and skullcaps bustled by. One stopped by my bed, checked the name and numbers on my wristband, and wheeled me into an operating room. I was lifted from my bed onto the narrow operating table.

"It's so narrow," I mumbled, thinking that my friend Hattie would never fit. "Don't some people fall off?"

"We have wider ones for wider people," a nearby voice answered.

Tubes and other apparatus were being positioned by the table. Gleaming instruments stood ready nearby. A giant-sized light hung suspended overhead.

A figure clad in green surgical clothes, a green skullcap, and a green face mask stood by my side. I recognized my doctor.

"Hi," I smiled up at him.

"Hi," he said, returning my smile. He put his hand across my body and patted me gently while we waited. I felt reassured. I was glad that I had chosen him.

"Will you do the operation?" I had asked him back in June. I knew that gynecologists do routine hysterectomies, but I didn't know if they operated on cancer patients.

The oncologist would do the surgery, he had answered. She was a top surgeon, this was her expertise, and I would be well taken care of.

"Could you do it?" I had pushed. "Do you do this kind of cancer surgery?"

He could do it, he had said, but she was my oncologist. He assured me that she could perform the surgery as well as he could; I didn't have to worry.

"I'd like you to do it," I had persisted. "If I have any choice at all, I want you to operate."

He had thought for a moment.

"If you want me to do it, I will," he had said. And he agreed to talk with my oncologist.

Why had I wanted him? I knew that my oncologist was tops, that patients came to her from all over the state, that she did this type of surgery more often than my gynecologist did. Still, I had wanted him. I had known him for fourteen years, I liked him, and I had confidence in him. He had delivered Jeffrey. No, he hadn't delivered Jeffrey. I had delivered Jeffrey by myself while he sat by my side.

"Why do you want to have natural childbirth?" he had asked me when he had confirmed my pregnancy more than ten years before. "We deliver hundreds of babies here and ninety-eight percent of the mothers take some kind of painkillers. It's much more pleasant—both for the mother and for the doctor."

But I had wanted natural childbirth. So we had discussed it and agreed that assuming a normal uncomplicated labor, he would give me no medication without my consent and knowledge. Giving birth to Jeffrey remains one of the most memorable experiences of my life.

Now I was on the operating table, prepped and draped in the usual sterile manner for a radical abdominal procedure. My surgeon stood over me, reassuringly. Somehow I knew that he cared about me.

"Oh God," I prayed, squeezing my eyes shut to hold back the tears. "Take care of me. Please take care of me."

"You'll go to sleep now," my doctor said gently. His voice sounded distant. "When you wake up, it'll be all over."

I felt myself losing consciousness. My head was swirling in a black void.

"Good night, Elaine," I heard faintly.

And then there was nothing.

* * *

For the next three days, I drifted in and out of consciousness. I slept, I woke, I slept again. Ralph was there, a nurse was there, maybe someone else. I didn't know.

The days were a fog of pain. I tried to focus, I tried to speak, but I kept dozing off. Everything was blurry. I was drugged at all times.

Tubes were attached to all parts of my body. I lay pale and listless; was I dead or alive? Around-the-clock nurses moistened my parched lips with ice chips.

My recovery was fragmented and barely real. As clarity increased, so did the pain. The pain reminded me that I was alive. I had not died on the operating table. I had survived the surgery.

Ralph, Debra, and Rachel had stayed in the waiting room, pacing back and forth and drinking coffee. Our Rabbi had joined them for a short while. After what had seemed to them like an eternity, my doctor came into the waiting room. They saw in an instant that he wore a smile.

"She's fine," he told my husband and children. "She's in the recovery room. We think we got it all."

Relief! Thankfulness! Release from tension! Tears of joy, hugs of happiness, prayers of thanks. His wife, their mother, would live.

* * *

The tumor was confined to my uterus. My uterus, ovaries and tubes had been removed, the surrounding area looked clean, and the adjacent lymph nodes had been removed as a precautionary measure. My surgeon hadn't opened up the uterus, so he couldn't determine what state the tumor was in, whether it was still there or whether it had been destroyed by the radiation. The whole organ had been sent to the laboratory for tests. We would have the results in about three days.

Everyone was optimistic. The operation was a success; everything was out. Things were going according to plan—chemotherapy, radiation, surgery. Now the surgery was finished, and I was on the road to recovery.

Rachel sat by my side. It was Friday morning, three days after the surgery, and I was still in pain. My doctor came in and sat down at the edge of my bed.

"Elaine," he said, "I have good news and I have bad news."

My fuzzy mind became alert, and I tried hard to concentrate.

"The good news is that we removed the tumor," he said. "It was confined to the uterus, and we found no indication of any cancer anyplace else."

He paused for a moment, giving me time to digest this information.

"The bad news," he continued, "is that when the uterus was opened up in the laboratory, they found that the tumor was still there. It was not destroyed as we hoped it would be; it was alive and still virulent."

I lay there speechless. I just looked at him.

"We're going to have to give you some more chemotherapy," he said gently.

"No!" I cried, rejecting the very idea. "I don't want any more chemotherapy. If the cancer is out of my body, what difference does it make how dead or alive it was. Just take the whole uterus and throw it out."

It wasn't so simple, he explained. Since the tumor was still active, there was a slight possibility that a few cells may have escaped during the surgery. Even if just one tiny microscopic cell was in my bloodstream, it could mean that the cancer might recur. He wanted to protect me against that possibility.

The implications of what he was telling me registered in my brain. So it wasn't over. I would need more chemotherapy, I would continue to feel lousy, and still I wouldn't know that I was safe. The worry, the uncertainty, the dread would continue. And the worst might still lie ahead.

"No!" I screamed silently! "No more! I can't stand any more." I turned my head into my pillow and cried uncontrollably.

Rachel didn't know how to comfort me. What could she do to change the way it was? What solace could she bring? How could she help make it easier for me?

The phone rang.

"Don't answer it," I sobbed, as Rachel reached for the phone. "I don't want to talk to anyone."

"Maybe it's Daddy," she said.

"Don't answer it," I insisted. "Let it ring."

I cried for a long time. I tried to think rationally, and the more I thought, the angrier I became. What's the purpose of all this stuff if it doesn't work, I wondered. I had been treated aggressively for four months and the tumor was still alive, virulent. So what good was the chemotherapy, the radiation, the implant? And what about my future? I wanted to resume a normal life. I wanted to be healthy, active, productive. Instead I was back where I was four months ago, miserable, with no end in sight. I had thought the surgery would be the end of my ordeal. Now I wondered if it was only the beginning.

The phone rang again.

"Don't answer it," I told Rachel.

"Maybe I should," she said. "Unless it's Daddy, I'll say that you're sleeping."

"Does Daddy know about this?" I asked Rachel.

"He knows," she said. "He spoke with the doctor this morning."

I picked up the phone and heard Ralph's voice.

"Where are you?" I screamed hysterically. "Why aren't you here? How could you go to work and leave me alone when you knew what the doctor would tell me? How come you're not here when I need you?"

Suddenly, I realized what I was saying. I stopped screaming and started crying again.

"I'm sorry," I cried into the phone. "I'm sorry, Ralph. I'm just so upset." Then I handed the phone to Rachel and cried harder.

I cried all morning. I felt helpless, and my situation seemed hopeless. How could I handle more chemotherapy? And so soon after major surgery. It wasn't fair. I wallowed in self-pity.

Chemotherapy would begin that very night. I would be given an overload dose of intravenous Cytoxan for five consecutive days. No one was wasting any time.

I learned later that chemotherapy had not been my doctors' first choice. My gynecologist and my oncologist had approached my radiotherapists to discuss post-operative radiation. "We can't," the radiotherapist had told them. "She's already had the maximum dosage. We can't give her any more." They had discussed alternatives and decided on Cytoxan.

I didn't want to be sick from the chemotherapy. My parents were coming on Sunday, and I didn't want them to see me in pain. But I had no control. I was sick on Friday night, sicker on Saturday night, and horribly sick on Sunday. I had nausea and vomiting, fever and chills, dizziness and drowziness, constant diarrhea, and hideous unrelenting abdominal cramps. And still the chemotherapy was administered regularly, every day at four o'clock. The entire scene was a horrible nightmare.

Sunday, August 10, was my birthday. I was forty-one years old.

* * *

My mother smiled and kissed me. She pulled a chair up to my bed and sat down. She did not cry.

My father planted a quick kiss on my head and left the room. It was a while before he came back, and when he did, his eyes were red.

I lay there encased in my white sheets, my rumpled scarf encircling my head. From the plastic bag hanging on the intravenous stand, purple blood dripped. It traveled down the plastic tube, passed through a blood warming machine, and entered my body through a vein in my lower arm. My parents had come during a blood transfusion.

My father was a big man, almost six feet tall, with a thick mop of white hair. He was knowledgeable and worldly, a self-starter, who from scratch had built up a successful business. But his biggest success—his pride and joy—had always been his three daughters. When we were children, he had played with us often, from piggy-back rides, to checkers, to gin rummy. As teenagers, we had spent countless hours talking and planning; planning our dates, our parties, and ultimately our weddings. He was so proud of us, our husbands, our children, and all our accomplishments. We had never disappointed him.

When my parents had last seen me in June, I had looked awful. My skin had been sallow, dark circles had surrounded my eyes, and I had been weak and chronically tired. It had been hard for them to deal with seeing me so sick. Now I looked so much worse, so much sicker, as I lay in the hospital bed hooked up to the intravenous apparatus. I had been waiting for my parents to arrive, listening intently to the footsteps in the corridor and hoping each time that it was them. I did not anticipate the effect that my appearance would have on them.

At four o'clock, the nurse arrived with my chemotherapy. My father, who was sitting near the wall, turned pale.

"Maybe you should go out, Daddy," I said. "You don't have to watch this."

"It's okay, it's okay," he said.

The nurse began feeding the chemotherapy into the intravenous unit. My father grew more and more pale. I thought he would faint before the first drop entered my veins. My mother got up, escorted him into the corridor, and told him not to come back in until she came to get him.

My mother was a petite woman. With her short back hair, slim figure, and crinkly eyes that seemed always to be smiling, she looked much younger than her years. I had always taken my mother for granted. Until now, I hadn't appreciated her strength.

My mother spent every day of the next two weeks in the hospital. She did exactly what I needed her to do. She brought me things when a nurse wasn't around, and sometimes she brought them when a nurse was around. She answered the phone and handled the calls I didn't feel well enough to take. She covered me with blankets when I had chills, and she removed them when I dripped with sweat. She brought me the bedpan, and she held a dishpan to my face when I needed to throw up. She brought my favorite foods, and she tried so hard to convince me to eat something. She talked to my doctors, she talked to me, and she listened to me. Throughout the haze of the pain, and the drugs, and the nurses, and the tubes, and the bandages, something was all right. My mother was there.

* * *

I sat in a chair and leaned my head against the wall. Under the blankets that were wrapped around me, my hands clutched my abdomen. It was eight days since my surgery, and I was still feeling weak and having abdominal pain. I waited for a nurse to come help my mother take me back to my bed.

A figure appeared in the doorway. I looked up and saw my friend Hattie.

"Hattie!" I said with surprise." "How did you get here?" "I walked," she answered.

"All by yourself?" I asked incredulously.

"Well, I had to hold on to the walls a little," she said.

I stared at her. Hattie had had surgery only three days ago. How did she walk down the hall from her room to mine? I couldn't walk, I couldn't even sit without pain, and I was already eight days postoperative.

"I can't walk yet," I said to Hattie. "I'm still so weak."

"That's because of all the poisons they're pumping into you," she told me. "I'm not getting any chemotherapy. You'll get stronger when the chemo wears off."

"Come in and sit down," my mother invited Hattie who was still standing in the doorway. She offered Hattie her chair.

"I better not," Hattie said. "I think I'll go back to my room before I get too tired. I'll come again though, and you come visit me when you can. I'm just a few doors down the hall."

Hattie walked back to her room unaided.

"It's not fair," I said to my mother. "I'm twenty years younger than she is, and look at her and look at me."

"She's bigger and stronger than you are," my mother answered. "And she's not taking chemotherapy. You'll get better too," she said reassuringly. "It may take a little longer, but you'll get better."

I was jealous of Hattie. I didn't want to be jealous, but I was. I wanted to walk too, I wanted not to have to take chemotherapy, I wanted my pain to go away, I wanted to go home. And I wanted my mother to see me well.

What would I do without my mother, I wondered. My mother was always there when I needed her. Would I always be there for my children, I wondered? Would they have the comfort of knowing that if ever they needed me, I'd be there? Or would my children not have a mother much longer? I rejected that possibility. I could not allow that to happen. I would get better. It might take a little longer, but I would get better. I would be a warm and loving mother again. I would give my children the gift that my mother had given me—the security of knowing that I would always be there when they needed me.

And I would regain my self-respect. From a happy, healthy, energetic, and stable woman, I had been reduced to a state of dependency, to constant tears, to a physical, mental, and emotional wreck. I was not a crier, I was not self-pitying, I was a giver and not a taker. More than anything, I wanted to go back to the way I was. I wanted to regain my dignity.

There was one thing I was determined to do before I left the hospital. My mother supported me on one side, a nurse supported me on the other side, and between them, I stumbled down the hall to visit Hattie.

* * *

When I had accepted a job as a business teacher, I hadn't known I would be taking chemotherapy. With my surgery scheduled for the first week in August, I had thought I would be able to recuperate over the summer and begin teaching in September. Now this was impossible. Reluctantly, I resigned from my job.

When the five days of intravenous chemotherapy were completed, I resumed taking Cytoxan and Megace orally, three times a day.

"How long will I have to take this?" I asked my oncologist.

Her answer startled me. "Perhaps up to two years," she said.

"Two years!" I repeated, not wanting to believe what I heard. "Why up to two years?"

She explained that cancer behaves in many ways. Some cancers grow slowly, reappearing many years after the original diagnosis. Other cancers are more aggressive; when they recur, it happens quickly. My tumor was a very aggressive one. When this type of tumor spreads, it usually does so in the first two years. More recurrences occur in the first year than in the second, and the most vulnerable time is the first six months. For the next few months, I would be monitored very carefully, with chest X-rays, liver scans, and bone scans. I learned that the most common sites of recurrence are the lungs, the liver, and the bones.

Back home again, I resumed my reading. I was becoming more and more knowledgeable about cancer. There was something I was picking up from my readings that no one ever talked about, the nutritional link between diet and disease. Certain foods, I learned, had cancer-promoting qualities, and certain foods were cancer inhibitors. Many people had used nutrition to aid in their recovery. Some people believed in vitamin A, some took megadoses of vitamin C, and many espoused the attributes of vitamin E and selenium. Every book I read recommended a diet that was low in fat, low in sugar, and high in fiber.

I had spent so much time in the hospital. Countless doctors had asked me a myriad of questions about my past. No one had ever asked me what I was eating.

I stopped reading about cancer and began to study nutrition. I became a health food nut. Red meat was replaced with chicken. Low fat milk, cottage cheese, and yogurt became family staples. A big raw salad accompanied every dinner, and snacks became fresh fruit and nut and seed mixtures. I drank coffee substitutes and herbal teas.

Despite my low sugar, low fat diet, and a limited appetite, I continued to gain weight. I suspected that the Megace, with its high hormone content, was the cause, and my readings confirmed my thoughts. I was taking two hundred and forty milligrams of Megace every day.

My fatigue did not lessen. Every afternoon I took a three hour nap, and right after dinner I was tired again. Even when I was awake, my mind was never really clear. A sharpness, an alertness, a clear unclouded perspective was lacking. It was as if a veil was hanging over me, as if I was living in a fog that I couldn't shake away.

Bald from chemotherapy, fat from hormones, lacking adequate physical mobility and mental clarity, depression overcame me often. Where was the young energetic woman who always wore a smile? Where was the mother who laughed with her children? Where was the college student who was mistaken for a teenager and asked for dates? Where was the woman who played bridge and tennis, and bicycled around the park in the spring, and went ice-skating every Sunday in the winter. Where was the woman who liked to sing?

"Come back," I begged of myself often. "Will the real Elaine Nussbaum please come back."

* * *

I couldn't reach Hattie. We spoke to each other regularly, and for the past two weeks no one had answered her phone. I was concerned.

I knew that Hattie had a cold. She had gone to a wedding recently, the place was air-conditioned, and she hadn't brought a sweater. She had caught a cold that she didn't seem able to shake.

"She probably went to visit her daughter," Ralph told me. "Don't worry."

Hattie did spend a lot of time with her daughter, sometimes visiting for a week or two at a time. But why didn't she tell me? Other times she would let me know if she would be away for more than a few days.

Maybe she couldn't reach me, I thought. I take the phone off the hook when I nap every afternoon, and Rhonda and Jeffrey use the phone a lot at night. Maybe she just couldn't get through. Still I worried and wished she would call.

One day she did.

"Hattie," I said when I heard her voice. "I've been trying to reach you."

"I know," she said. "You couldn't reach me because I'm not where I'm supposed to be."

"Where are you?" I asked.

"In the hospital," she answered.

"In the hospital!" I repeated. "Why! What happened?"

Hattie had gone to the doctor to see if he could do anything for her cold. The doctor had detected fluid in her lungs, and Hattie had gone to the hospital to have the fluid drained. Testing of the fluid revealed that cancer cells were there.

I was speechless. What could I say? How could this be happening? Hattie was so strong. Look how quickly she bounced back from her implant, how fast she recovered from surgery. And her cancer wasn't virulent. She didn't even need chemotherapy. How could it have spread to her lungs?

"It's not a solid tumor," Hattie told me, "so I won't be having surgery. I'm just going to have some radiation."

I shuddered. The thought of lung surgery conjured up an image of my other roommate, who had suffered terribly and finally died.

"I'm glad it's not a solid tumor," I told Hattie. "Radiation's not nearly as bad as surgery. Some people don't have any side effects at all."

We talked a while longer, and Hattie promised to let me know how she was doing.

The radiation did not stop the cancer. Hattie got progressively worse, the cancer spreading throughout her body. She died in November, a few days before Thanksgiving.

Hattie's death had a devastating effect on me. I never felt more vulnerable. I'll die, too, I thought. Soon it will be my turn. The cancer always wins.

Or does it, I wondered. Some people survive cancer. Maybe I'll be the lucky one. Maybe I'll be the one to live.

My emotions were all confused. When I thought about my cancer friends who had died, I became depressed. When I thought of myself as the survivor, I was optimistic. My moods changed with my changing thoughts. And I couldn't stop thinking about Hattie.

"Is there anything I can do?" I asked her daughter.

"Remember her, Elaine," she asked of me. "She would want you to remember her."

"I will," I promised.

I will always remember my friend Hattie.

* * *

The cloud lifted, the fog disappeared, and I began to think clearly. I felt alive. My oncologist had advised me to stop taking the Cytoxan for two weeks. Regular check-ups had showed that I was not healing internally from the surgery, and she suspected that the Cytoxan was impeding the healing process.

"Can you manage one day without your nap?" Shayndee asked me.

"I can try," I answered. "Why?"

"I'll take a day off from work and take you out," she suggested.

Shayndee picked me up and we drove into New York. We went out for lunch and then to the theater. I came home both exhausted and exhilarated. It was a wonderful day, the nicest I had in a very long time.

Phyllis volunteered a day the next week.

"What would you like to do?" She asked me.

"Let's go shopping," I suggested.

We went to a shopping mall where we shopped, had a leisurely lunch, and shopped again until I got tired. We bought presents for the children for the approaching Chanukah holiday, and we bought a gift for my parents. Another wonderful day.

All too soon, my two week reprieve was over. I didn't want to resume the chemotherapy. And yet, I felt uneasy about not taking it. I felt unprotected, naked, vulnerable. What a choice; to feel better and vulnerable or to feel lousy and safer!

My check-up revealed that I was starting to heal. I was given another reprieve.

I was able to attend our annual family Chanukah party. The Chanukah holiday lasts eight days, and a family celebration on the Sunday of Chanukah was a family tradition. We had dinner together, we lit candles, we sang songs, and we gave gifts to the children. Except for the times when one of the children was studying in Israel, no one had ever missed a Chanukah party.

There were twenty of us: Shayndee and Dani and their four children, Phyllis and Dave and their four children, the six of us, and my parents. All of us singing together around the

brightly lit candles was an overwhelmingly emotional experience. I buried my face in my hands and tried to muffle my
sobs. Would this be my last Chanukah?

Phyllis put her arm around me. She continued to sing
though her voice was shaky. Shayndee sang louder, trying
to keep the younger children's attention on the songs. No
one mentioned my breakdown. It wasn't necessary.

My next check-up showed that I was healing nicely. My
oncologist told me that I would not have to resume the
Cytoxan.

No more dull mind. No more depressed blood levels. No
more chronic fatigue and weakness and sleeping away each
day. Maybe my hair would even grow back. I would have
liked to stop taking the Megace too, but my oncologist
insisted that I continue. I didn't argue. Megace wasn't
debilitating. I would be able to function.

I returned to the hospital regularly for tests. Chest X-rays,
bone scans, and ultrasound scans of the pelvis continued to
come back negative. I was feeling better. I was on my way.

* * *

We sat on the wooden bench in the waiting room of the
nuclear medicine department. A liver scan had just been
taken, and I was told to wait until the doctor made sure that
the pictures were clear. Phyllis and I talked about where we
would go for lunch.

"Elaine Nussbaum?" a nurse asked me.

"Yes," I answered. "Can I leave now?"

"Not yet," was her reply. "The doctor would like some
more pictures."

My stomach turned queasy, and my legs felt weak.

"Why?" I asked.

"We need some larger pictures," she said, "and the doctor
would like a few from another angle. Come with me."

"Is anything wrong?" I stammered, as I followed her into

the scanning room, leaving a pale Phyllis behind. "Did anything show up on my pictures?"

"The pictures weren't clear," she answered. "We'll repeat some and just take a few new ones. It won't take long."

That's it, I thought to myself. The cancer spread to my liver. Otherwise, why would the doctor want more pictures? And why would he want to repeat the same ones if not to confirm that something was there?

This time, the nurse stayed in the room and advised the technician of the exact positions that the doctor wanted. I did not look at the screen. I was afraid I might see something I didn't want to see.

I rejoined Phyllis on the wooden bench and we waited. All kinds of thoughts jumped around in my mind. I tried not to cry.

"Are you all right?" asked the nurse when she reappeared. "Do you want some water?"

"I'm a cancer patient," I told her, trying to maintain some composure, "and I think it has spread to my liver. Could you tell me if any cancer showed up on these pictures?"

"Your doctor will tell you the results of the tests," she said.

"When will she know?" I asked.

"She'll have the report tomorrow. It's all right for you to leave now."

Phyllis and I didn't go out for lunch. Neither of us was hungry.

I called my oncologist early the next morning. Her nurse told me that the results hadn't come up yet.

"Could you call me as soon as you know?" I asked her. "I'm really nervous."

The nurse offered to call the nuclear medicine department and ask that they send up my report right away. As soon as the doctor reviewed it, she would call me back.

I glued myself to the phone. Each time it rang, fear and apprehension welled up inside me. Ralph called, and the children, and Shayndee, and Phyllis, and some friends.

"No news yet," I said to my family. "Can't talk now," I said to my friends. And I sat by the phone and waited.

By one o'clock I was frantic. It was Friday, and I knew that unless I found out this afternoon, I would have to wait until Monday. There was no way I could get through the weekend like this.

I called the hospital. The line was busy. How can a hospital's line be busy?

I dialed again.

"Hospital. Will you hold, please?" a voice said, and she was gone before I could answer.

I sat in helpless silence on hold. I thought about hanging up, but I knew that I wouldn't. Finally, the voice returned. "May I help you?"

"Yes," I said. I asked to be connected with my oncologist's office.

"Hold please," she left me again. A few minutes passed.

"Doctor's office," said a new voice. "Just a minute please." And I was left on hold again.

"May I help you?" asked the nurse.

"It's Elaine Nussbaum again," I said. "Is there any news on my liver scan."

"I think the report came up," she said. "Just a minute and I'll check."

A few minutes passed and she was back.

"Elaine," she said. "Your liver scan is fine."

"Thank you," I said, and tears of relief streamed freely down my face. My liver was fine.

On Monday I called the nurse again.

"I wonder if you can tell me," I asked her, "why my liver scan had to be repeated?"

She didn't know, but she would try to find out.

And she did.

The nuclear medicine department was training a new technician. This student-technician did not have me positioned properly for the scan, nor did she focus the machine correctly for clear pictures. So the procedure had to be repeated under the direction of a qualified nurse.

Why hadn't the nurse told me why the pictures were unclear? She had seen my fright, my anguish, and she had offered me a glass of water to pacify me. Where was some sensitivity for the feelings of the patient?

It was one year after my surgery and my tests were all negative. A box from Phyllis arrived in the mail. It contained a single rose. "Happy Anniversary!" the card read. "Next year I'll send you two."

* * *

With Debra and Rachel holding full time summer jobs, and Rhonda and Jeffrey back in overnight camp, I needed something to do for the summer. I took a part-time job in a health food store.

I worked two days a week from ten o'clock until two o'clock with a twenty minute break for lunch. I was paid an hourly wage plus commission, and I received a discount on my personal shopping. Most of my salary went back to the store in the form of purchases of peanut butter, yogurt, dried fruits, nuts and seeds, herbal teas, honey, and vitamins. I bought bread without preservatives, cheese without rennet, and eggs that were laid by free-roaming chickens that hadn't been debeaked. I liked the job, and I got home early enough to take a nap before dinner.

One day each week, and sometimes two, I spent with Shayndee. We went to the beach, to the park, to the theater, to a blueberry festival, to a shopping mall, to the beach again. One day we stayed home and made apple strudel. Another day we made stuffed cabbage. Shayndee arrived with some oversized pots and twenty-seven pounds of cabbage which we stuffed with twenty pounds of chopped meat. We used honey instead of sugar, and the eggs came from free-roaming chickens. At the end of an exhausting day, we had one hundred and forty cabbage rolls, which we stashed away in our freezers in anticipation of the forthcoming holidays.

Shayndee did a lot of driving, as it is a forty-minute ride from her house to mine, and I pushed myself, sometimes to the point of exhaustion. But we enjoyed and cherished the time we spent together. It was a good summer.

In the fall, I increased my work time to three days a week, and I often did substitute teaching on the other days. I continued my periodic X-rays, my Megace, my daily naps, and my study of nutrition. I read every nutrition book in the library, and I bought the books that the library didn't have. When I had exhausted my supply of reading materials, I enrolled in school again and began taking courses towards a master's degree in nutrition.

In June 1982, Ralph and I celebrated our twenty-fifth wedding anniversary. The children, with the help of Shayndee and Phyllis, hosted a gala surprise party for us in Shayndee's backyard. My parents came from Florida, Ralph's mother, his brother Jack and sister Naomi were there, and his brother Mike flew in from Chicago. In addition to the platters of food that they ordered, Debra and Rachel prepared a variety of health salads, and Debra went through my recipe box and baked some of my favorite natural cookies and cakes. It was a wonderful party, a wonderful day. I even forgot about the intermittent pain that I was having in my lower back.

*　*　*

Chapter 4

IT WAS A DULL ACHE, A THROBBING, just enough to keep me aware of the fact that I had a back. It started in May and gradually intensified, and by the end of June the pain was constant.

"Don't worry," I told myself. "Everyone has lower back pain sometimes. It'll go away."

Ralph wanted me to see a doctor.

"Who?" I asked him. "I can't bother my oncologist with an aching back."

"What about an orthopedist?" Ralph suggested.

I refused. I didn't want to get involved with any new doctors. Not now. It was almost two years since my surgery, and with each passing month I felt surer and surer that my cancer wouldn't recur. In August I would be forty-three. Forty-three and cancer free had become my goal. And now I was just a few weeks away from reaching it. I would wait until August for my clean bill of health. Then, if my back still bothered me, I would get it checked out.

The pain didn't abate, and a gnawing fear started growing inside me.

"What does an oncologist know about backs, anyway?" I challenged Ralph, who was getting more and more persistent that I see someone.

"Then see a chiropractor," Ralph suggested. "He helped me, remember?"

I remembered. Three years earlier, Ralph had hurt his back putting up storm windows. He had seen an orthopedist who had prescribed medication and recommended bed rest. It hadn't helped. Ralph then saw another orthopedist who prescribed different medication and more bed rest. That hadn't helped either. Ralph had lain in bed for four weeks, and finally, in desperation, had called a chiropractor. After the first session with the chiropractor, he had been able to walk a little without pain. He had continued seeing the chiropractor, had gotten progressively better, and the pain had never recurred.

I agreed to see the chiropractor.

Because of my previous history of cancer, the chiropractor recommended that I have X-rays taken. The X-rays showed a slight density on my lower spine.

"What does it mean?" I asked him, trying to suppress the rising fear.

He said that it was probably nothing serious, but he thought I should contact my oncologist to see if she wanted to check it out.

I called my oncologist, and we scheduled a bone scan for July 28.

Now I was really scared. The pain was becoming increasingly stronger. I couldn't sit in a soft chair, and it was painful for me to get in and out of a car. We bought a lumbosacral belt which I wore all day, and I started doing exercises specifically for lower back pain. We tried to make my sleep more comfortable by putting a wooden board under my mattress. Nothing helped. The pain kept getting worse. I started sleeping on the floor.

Rhonda was a counselor in overnight summer camp, and Jeffrey was a camper there. By visiting day, which was the third Sunday in July, I couldn't sit at all. Ralph padded the back of our station wagon with blankets, and I rode up to camp lying on my side, surrounded by pillows and bags of snacks for Rhonda and Jeffrey.

This couldn't be a recurrence of the cancer, I told myself. The timing is all wrong. My type of cancer spreads fast, usually within the first year, and only very rarely after two

years have passed. And it was just about two years from the
time of my surgery. If I count from the time of the diagnosis,
I told myself, then it's already two years and three months.
And besides, I ate so well. I made my own yogurt and fortified it with non-fat dry milk. I ate cottage cheese and Swiss
cheese regularly. Surely I had plenty of calcium. Every morning I had a fresh orange for vitamin C, every lunch included
an apple for fiber, and every day I had a banana for potassium. I loved bananas. Some days I even have two. Except
for liver, which I ate once a week for iron, I had no red meat,
and I always removed the skin from my chicken. I ate a raw
salad every day, I snacked on raw nuts and seeds, and I
sprouted alfalfa and mung beans. When I baked, I used whole
wheat flour instead of white, honey instead of sugar, and carob
instead of chocolate. My peanut butter was ground fresh in the
health food store. I took a multi-vitamin pill every morning,
I never forgot, and every night I took vitamin C. I was a
health food nut, a budding nutritionist. How could I have
cancer again?

On July 28, 1982, following an injection of radioactive dye,
I was imaged from my head to my feet in both the anterior
and posterior projections. Two days later, scared and in pain,
I went with Ralph to my oncologist for the results of the bone
scan.

She was behind in her schedule, and other patients were
ahead of us. We waited a long time in the waiting room.
Ralph sat, and I paced up and down. Finally, we were ushered
into the office.

"You have a fracture," my oncologist said as we walked
in the door. "A compression fracture of the spine."

"A fracture!" I repeated. "It's only a fracture!" I felt
tremendous relief as the tension left my body and I was
released from my gripping fear.

"It's a fracture!" I said again, happily turning to Ralph.
"I have a compression fracture!"

There was no treatment for my fracture, my oncologist told us. It would get better by itself in time. Meanwhile, I should try to be as active as possible.

"Does this have anything to do with the previous cancer?" Ralph asked.

"Not that we can see," was her answer.

We went home in a state of euphoria. There was no cancer. It was only a fracture! It hurt plenty, but I knew that fractures could be very painful. I could take the pain if I knew that it was only a fracture, that it would heal by itself, that it was not cancer. I needed only to be patient.

Rachel was waiting for us in front of the house.

"It's a fracture, Rach," I called to her even before Ralph stopped the car. "It's only a fracture!"

Rachel hugged me, she hugged Ralph, and she asked us to tell her exactly what the doctor had said. Rachel prepared a special supper while I called the family.

I dialed Shayndee. There was no answer. Where was Shayndee? She knew I had a four o'clock appointment. She had told me to call as soon as I got home, no matter what the diagnosis. Besides, it was suppertime. Why wasn't Shayndee home?

I dialed Phyllis. She picked up the phone the second it started to ring.

"It's not cancer, Phyl," I said happily. "It's a fracture. I have a fractured spine!"

"A fractured spine!" she exclaimed. "A fractured spine! Oh Elaine, I'm so happy. I'm so happy you have a fractured spine!"

We talked for a few minutes about how happy we were.

"Did you call Shayndee?" Phyllis asked.

"There's no answer," I said. "Where is she?"

"In the office," said Phyllis. "She didn't want to go home until she heard from you. She didn't want to break down in front of the kids if the news was bad. She wanted to be alone until she knew."

I called Shayndee at her office.

"Hello," said a shaky voice.

"It's not cancer, Shayn," I said. "It's a fracture. I have a fractured spine!"

Shayndee started to cry. "Thank God," she sobbed into the phone. "Thank God it's a fractured spine." Then she was laughing and crying at the same time. "I can't believe I'm thanking God that you have a fractured spine."

We called Rhonda and Jeffrey in camp, and we called my parents in Florida. We called Ralph's family in New York, and we called his brother Mike in Chicago. I called my friends. I was so happy, so relieved. I didn't have cancer. I had a fractured spine!

That night I wrote a long letter to Debra. Debra was studying in Israel for the summer, and although my back was already hurting when she left, we never wrote her about how severe the pain had become and about how worried we were. Now I wrote that I had had a bone scan, that the scan showed that there was no sign of cancer, but that I had a compression fracture of the spine. "Everything's fine," I wrote. "It will heal by itself and the pain will go away. It's only a fracture."

A floral arrangement arrived the next day. It was from Phyllis. "Dear Elaine," the card read, "Congratulations on your fracture."

On August 5, exactly two years after my surgery, another box arrived from Phyllis. Inside were two roses. The card read simply, "That's Two!"

*　　*　　*

The pain got worse. I couldn't sit, and I couldn't lie flat. I was standing up all day, and at night I slept on the hard floor with pillows under my knees. Sometimes I tried to raise my legs onto a chair or onto the bed to further relieve the pressure on my back. I slept on the floor a few hours, got up and walked a few hours, and then got back on the floor again and tried to sleep a little until morning. Ralph bought me a new mattress, a super firm one. I couldn't lie on it.

It was painful for me to bend. Getting down on the floor became an ordeal, and it was agony when I had to get up again. It wasn't long before the short time I could stay down was not worth the effort and the pain of getting there. I stood up all day and all night.

Ralph would wake up in the middle of the night and find me in the kitchen, leaning on the counter and reading a nutrition book. Or I would be backed into a corner, holding on to a chair and trying to doze a little. Sometimes Ralph stood by the wall, his arms around me, and I would rest my head on his shoulder and sleep. For four days, I neither sat nor lay down.

I called the hospital. There was no point in taking more X-rays or bone scans, I was told. I would have to wait at least two months after the previous series, otherwise the results would almost certainly be the same as before.

I called an orthopedist. I was given an appointment for three weeks later.

"I'm in terrible pain," I said to the nurse. "I can't sit or lie down. Could you possibly squeeze me in sooner?"

She said that she couldn't.

The orthopedist was one of a team of three. "Can I see one of the other doctors?" I pleaded. "I'll see any doctor, and I'll come any time of the day or night. I need to see someone soon."

"I'm sorry, that's the earliest I can give you," she sounded annoyed. "Do you want the appointment?"

I took it, and I asked her to please call me if she had a cancellation before that.

A good friend, a practicing physiotherapist, recommended another orthopedist, who was head of orthopedic surgery at the hospital where I was being treated. Ralph had developed a regular dialogue with our physiotherapist/friend. In addition to freely answering questions about my illness and treatment, he had prescribed a number of surgical supplies which were extremely helpful in my painful condition. Now we called the orthopedist he recommended.

The nurse gave me an appointment for the following week.

"I'm in terrible pain," I told her. "Could he possibly see me sooner? I'll come any time of the day or night."

"Just a minute, please," she clicked off, and she returned a few minutes later.

"The doctor will see you tomorrow morning," she said. I thanked her profusely.

The waiting room was full. There were people with broken arms, broken legs, broken toes, and aching backs. Everyone was sitting. I paced back and forth.

"Why don't you have a seat, Mrs. Nussbaum?" the nurse asked. "It may be a while."

"I can't sit," I told her. I continued to pace back and forth while the other patients stared at me with pity. "I can't sit," I explained to them as I passed. "And it's easier for me to walk than to stand still."

Finally my turn came. I couldn't get up on the examining table.

"How long has your back been hurting?" the doctor asked me, as he examined me standing up.

I gave him a brief summary of my cancer and my fracture. He asked a lot of questions. He seemed concerned, sympathetic, caring. I liked him.

"I'd like to look at your X-rays," he said, when he finished examining me.

The nurse requisitioned my X-rays, and I paced again in the waiting room while he studied them.

Back in the examining room, the orthopedist confirmed the compression fracture. He told me that in addition to the fracture, I had a partially collapsed vertebra.

"What does that mean?" I asked.

He explained that my backbone was collapsing. When the collapsing bone presses against other bone and surrounding nerves, pain results. He recommended a brace. The brace would hold the bone straight and keep it from pressing on the nerves. Hopefully, this would reduce the pain. We would try to prevent a total collapse of my vertebrae, he told me.

He prescribed Motrin to be taken on a regular basis for the pain. He also gave me a prescription for Fiorinol with codeine that I could take if the pain would become severe. He measured me for the brace, recommended a place where I could have it made up, and asked me to come back so that he could make sure that the fit was right for me. He would call my oncologist and advise her of my visit and his recommendations.

It was called a Jewitt Expansion Brace. It began just below the front of my neck and came down below my abdomen. A thick padding wrapped around my back, and steel rods extended down my sides. A heavy bar ran across my chest and another ran across my belly. The brace opened to be wrapped around me, and after it was fastened I was to screw it on very tight, as tight as I could stand it. I was screwed into a vise.

The orthopedist approved the brace. He recommended that I wear a cotton tee shirt underneath it to minimize irritation to my skin. I was to wear it always—twenty-four hours a day.

The pressure was constant. The bar across my chest felt as if a ton of bricks was sitting on me. The bar across my stomach felt like a girdle that was too tight. The thick padding around my back felt like my back was being pushed to my front. The pain was still there, but for the first few days it seemed more bearable.

Then it mounted again, increasing daily, and it wasn't long before it surpassed what it had been before. I began to have spasms, usually during the night. The pain would intensify, build up to a peak, and hold me in an excruciating unbearable state before it would slowly diminish. The spasms were coming two or three times a night, cramping, kinking, piercing pain that had me crying, pleading, begging for release.

"Oh God, make it go away," I cried. "Take it away. I can't stand any more."

I was taking Motrin three times a day. It did nothing. I

found that when I took the Fiorinal, forty-five minutes later I would get some relief. The relief lasted about two hours. I found myself counting how many hours I could go without Fiorinal. The interval between pills got shorter and shorter. I was taking more and more Fiorinal until I realized that it wasn't helping anymore. The pain was constant, the spasms continued.

Another problem developed. I was getting stomach-aches. Every few hours I would experience sharp, piercing pain in my stomach. Sometimes the stomach pain exceeded the back pain. During one agonizing stomach seizure, Ralph picked me up, put me in the back of our station wagon, and took me to the hospital emergency room. The resident who examined me recommended that I stop the Fiorinal. He prescribed Tylenol with codeine instead.

I finished the Motrin and didn't renew it. I stopped the Fiorinal and took the Tylenol instead. The stomach seizures kept coming.

I called the orthopedist. "Could the stomach seizures be caused by the pressure of the brace?" I asked him. He didn't think so. In his many years of practice, he had never found a brace to cause stomach problems. I called the man who fitted the brace. "Impossible," he said. "The brace couldn't possibly be the cause." I called my oncologist. She was away. I called a gastroenterologist.

The gastroenterologist was a personal friend. He was a top specialist with a busy practice, yet he always had time for us when we had a question. When my cancer had been first diagnosed, Ralph had asked his advice about moving me to another hospital, getting a second opinion, the competence of my doctors, the accuracy of my protocol, the effects of the treatments, and a myriad of other considerations. When I had been in the hospital for my surgery, he had come every morning to check on me. He had conferred with my doctors, he had talked with my mother, with Ralph, and with me. It had been comforting to know that he was there if I needed him. I tried not to abuse the privilege of our friendship.

Now I called him professionally. His nurse told me that he did not have office hours tomorrow, and that he was filled up for the rest of the week. I made an appointment for the following week and I asked the nurse to please let him know that I had called for an appointment.

Less than half an hour later, the nurse called back. The doctor had called in, and he would come to the office to see me tomorrow morning.

"Can you take the brace off so I can examine you?" he asked me when we arrived at his office.

Ralph unfastened the brace, and the doctor, the nurse, and Ralph helped me onto the examining table. I couldn't lie flat, so pillows were put under my head, my upper back, and my knees.

Then a strange thing happened. My stomach stopped hurting. Wherever he pressed, it didn't hurt. I felt silly. Where was the pain? My back throbbed. I couldn't turn or move without back pain, but my stomach felt fine.

The doctor completed his examination. There was no obstruction, he assured me, no tenderness, nothing that could account for the severe pain I was having. There was nothing wrong with my stomach.

"Have you been able to lie like this without stomach pain before?" he asked me.

"No," I told him. "I can't lie down at all."

"When did the pain begin?" he asked.

I wasn't sure of the exact date, I told him. It came on gradually.

"Did it start after you put on the brace?" he asked.

I was sure that it had.

Well I wasn't wearing the brace right now, we agreed. This was the first time I took off the brace, and it was the first time the stomach pain subsided. He felt that the brace, with the constant pressure of the bar across my stomach, was very likely the cause of my pain. He recommended an adjustment of the brace to relieve the pressure on my stomach.

Ralph locked me into the brace again, and he and the doctor went back into the office. The nurse stayed in the examining room to finish dressing me.

"How much does she know?" the doctor asked Ralph.

"Everything," Ralph told him. "We decided to be open and honest. No secrets. She wants to know, she needs to know. I haven't concealed anything."

I came into the office. "Sit down and we'll talk," the doctor said.

"I can't," I told him. "I can't sit."

"This feels very strange," he said. "I'm sitting behind my desk and you're standing in front of it."

"You should see us at dinner," Ralph volunteered. "I sit and she eats standing up."

We made some small talk and then got to the point. My gastroenterologist/friend had spoken to my doctors, and he had also conferred with some other specialists. They had reviewed my records and my scans; there was no sign of malignancy. However, sometimes cancer doesn't show up on a bone scan until a certain amount of degeneration has already taken place. We could not rule out that possibility.

"Do you think it's cancer?" I asked.

He told me that bone pain doesn't always mean cancer. It could mean anything—fracture, calcification, osteoporosis, discs, nerves, and he mentioned some other possibilities. Time was on my side, he reminded me. My type of cancer usually spreads in the first year, and it was now more than two years since my diagnosis. And I looked good. Some cancer patients have a certain look about them that says "cancer." I didn't have it. He said that hopefully it wasn't cancer, but that we couldn't discount the possibility.

"If it is," I asked him, "do you know how I'll be treated?"

He told me that my oncologist would decide, but he felt certain that I would be given radiation to alleviate the pain.

I didn't want to think about radiation. Or about cancer. I had a fracture and a partially collapsed vertebra. That's what my X-rays showed. A fracture is painful, a collapsing backbone is painful, and I had both, so of course I was in a lot of pain. A fracture does not mean cancer, back pain does not mean cancer, there was no reason for me to believe that I might have cancer.

My next X-rays and bone scan were scheduled for September 28. It was only a week away.

*   *   *

"If I lower the bar," the brace fitter told me on the phone, "you won't be able to sit."

"That's okay," I said. "I can't sit anyway."

"You don't understand," he said. "You won't be able to sit at all."

I assured him that I understood, and that being unable to sit was not the issue. The pressure had to be removed from my belly. My doctor said so, I told him.

He agreed to lower the bar so that it wouldn't press against my stomach.

As there was no way I could make the trip, Ralph took the brace while I stood leaning on the kitchen counter, waiting.

The bar ran across my pelvis. The stomach pain receded, never to return.

There was no relief from the back pain. I took Tylenol with codeine every three hours, and sometimes I took two at a time. Sometimes I wanted to swallow the whole bottle. The spasms continued, hideous unrelenting pain that gripped me and wouldn't let go. It was no longer confined to my lower back. The pain was reaching out, extending to my middle back, my thighs, my buttocks. It spread to my legs, piercing pain shooting down the front of my legs and around the back to my calves. My pain-wracked legs could no longer support me. I crumbled; I could no longer stand.

I couldn't sit, I couldn't stand, I couldn't lie down. Ralph put me into his reclining chair.

The chair had been a gift for Ralph on his fortieth birthday from the children and me. It had been delivered on his birthday, we had covered it with a big sheet, and we had waited impatiently for him to come home from work.

"What's that?" he had asked when he saw the sheet in the middle of the living room.

"It's for you!" we had told him excitedly. "Look and see!"

"Surprise!" we had shouted as he removed the sheet. And then we had all sung "Happy Birthday."

Now, seven years later, Ralph placed me in the chair in the semi-reclining position, and there I stayed, popping my pills.

Monday, September 27, the day before my scheduled X-rays and bone scan, was Yom Kippur, the most solemn of the Jewish holidays, a day of prayer and fasting. I fasted and prayed all day. This was my last chance. Today would determine my fate. I prayed to God to be kind, to have mercy, to take pity on me and my family. I prayed that my family be spared the anguish of watching me die a slow, agonizing, terribly painful death from cancer. I made bargains and promises, I atoned for my sins, I pleaded, I begged for mercy and forgiveness, I prayed for my life. All day, I stayed in my special chair and prayed.

Ralph and the children spent the day in the Synagogue. They took turns coming home to stay with me. My husband, my children, my parents, my sisters and my friends— everyone prayed for my recovery. Surely God was listening. He was kind and just. Surely He would hear our prayers and grant me life.

On Tuesday, September 28, I fortified myself with pain-killers for the ten-minute drive to the hospital. Ralph removed my brace, and he and the technician carefully lifted me onto the scanning table. The machine clicked on.

My two years of waiting were over. Now we would know.

* * *

So much had happened in the last two years, so many changes in our family life. Debra had completed an MSW, a master's degree in social work, and now she was working part-time while looking for a full-time position. Rachel had graduated from New York University with a degree in special education, and she had recently accepted a job with the bank where she had worked part-time as a student. Both Debra and Rachel had studied in Israel, and Rhonda had recently left to spend her first year of college there.

We had made plans for Jeffrey's Bar-Mitzvah, which would be in February 1983, on the holiday of Purim. Jeffrey was preparing to read the Megillah, the Book of Esther, at our Synagogue, and we had planned to follow the service with a reception in his honor. Now we had no idea what my condition would be like; in five months I might be healed of my fracture or I might be dying of cancer.

Since we had not been able to move to California, Ralph had been working in his company's Development Division. He had requested to be considered for an assignment in an operating division, and in early September 1982, an offer had been made. Ralph considered it to be an excellent opportunity and a great challenge, as it was considered a high growth area for the company. The job required a lot of direct attention, and it involved domestic business and world-wide planning responsibilities. Ralph was looking forward to getting totally immersed in this new position. It was exactly what he had been looking for for many years, and he was anxious to do a good job.

Ralph tried to maintain a balance between home and job responsibilities. His new position required time, dedication, and concentration, and I was requiring more and more time and attention as I became less and less self-sufficient. Ralph was working on an important project which had to be completed by mid-October. His work load had become overwhelming.

My parents wanted to help. They decided to come in October to help care for me so that Ralph could go to work and get some sleep. They would stay a few weeks, until I got back on my feet again.

Now we were all nervously awaiting the results of my X-rays and bone scan.

* * *

We wouldn't have the results of my tests until my next appointment with my oncologist, which was scheduled for Monday, October 4, almost a week away. Ralph asked our gastroenterologist/friend if he could find out sooner and let us know.

All day Wednesday, the day after the tests, I waited for him to call. A dozen times, I almost phoned him. Don't be a pest, I told myself. When he knows, he'll call.

By Thursday I couldn't stand the waiting. I phoned his office and asked that he call me back.

I waited. The phone finally rang. It was Ralph.

"Ralph," I said. "We can't tie up the phone." I told him that I called the doctor and I was waiting for him to return the call.

"I know," Ralph said. "I just spoke to him."

"What happened?" I asked.

The doctor had been in the hospital with my records. He had phoned his office and his nurse told him that I had called. Before returning my call, he had phoned Ralph at work.

He had told Ralph the results of my X-rays and scan.

"Don't call her back," Ralph had said to him. "I'll tell her."

* * *

Every glimmer of hope vanished. The phone fell from my hand, and the tears came.

"Are you all right?" I heard Ralph's voice from the dangling phone.

"No," I sobbed.

"Should I come home?"

Dumb question. Why hadn't he just come home instead of telling me on the phone. I didn't answer.

"I'm leaving right now," he said.

He found me in the chair, dissolved in tears. He took me in his arms, and we cried together.

The cancer was in my bones. There was also a mass in my lung. We were defeated. The cancer had won.

* * *

"We have a little setback," my oncologist said.

I sat slouched in a wheelchair, and Ralph held my hand. We had come to the hospital to discuss my X-rays and bone scan and my future treatments. A hospital attendant had helped Ralph lift me into a wheelchair.

My oncologist had planned immediate chemotherapy for me, but one look at my condition convinced her that I wouldn't be able to withstand it. She decided on radiation first, a palliative measure, an attempt to reduce the pain.

I would be given ten radiation treatments to the back. It would be a split series, five treatments now and another five next month. I would also have ten cycles of chemotherapy. Chemotherapy would be given every three to four weeks, and each cycle would require an overnight stay in the hospital. My chemotherapy would consist of Adriamycin and CCNU. We would begin my program tomorrow.

The next day, Tuesday October 5, Ralph took me back to the hospital for a planning session with the radiotherapy department. I took two painkillers before we left the house, two more when we got to the hospital, and when my turn with the radiotherapist came I needed two more. I could not lie on the X-ray table; the pain was excruciating. Neither could I lie down or sit to have my back marked. Ralph and a nurse had to hold me up while the radiotherapist drew his lines and boxes on my back with his purple marker. Ralph

had my pills in his pocket and I kept begging him for more.
I didn't care how many I took; I just wanted relief from the
horrible pain.

My treatments began the following day. My parents had
come the night before, and my mother joined us for the trip
to the hospital. She and Ralph managed to get me into a
wheelchair and wheel me to the radiation area. Into the treatment room they wheeled me, right up to the cot that stood
underneath the cobalt machine. Ralph and two technicians
held me up, while my mother removed my blouse and my
brace. Carefully, they lifted me and positioned me under the
machine. I had to lie on my stomach. It was the most horrible, hideous pain I had ever felt in my forty-three years of
life. I was given four hundred rads of cobalt, and the treatment lasted three minutes and forty-six seconds. I did not
think I would survive that long; I was sure I would die from
the pain before three minutes were up.

The technicians assured me that the pain would recede after
the first few treatments. I needed more than promises, I
needed some relief. I couldn't go on.

Ralph and my mother spoke with the head radiotherapist.
He prescribed Levo Dromamine.

Ralph couldn't get it. Pharmacy after pharmacy didn't
stock it. "That's narcotics," one pharmacist told Ralph.
"That's hard drugs," said another. Ralph called every drug
store in the telephone book until he found a pharmacist who
would get it for us.

On Friday, Ralph came home with the Levo Dromamine.
Warnings and precautions were written all over the label.
I took one. Nothing happened. The pain came right through.

On Saturday morning I took two together. The room
started moving. The pictures on the wall began dancing, my
eyes couldn't focus, everything was a blur. Green water came
gushing down the corners of the room, and the walls glistened
with streaks of silver-green drippings. Little elves with
brown paper bags over their heads came dancing into the
room. In single file they danced, jumped, and clapped,

and then they all joined hands and danced around in a circle. As the room swayed and the elves danced, I was transported out of my body, beyond pain, to a world of light and brilliant color. I was hallucinating.

As my eyes tried to focus, as my mind began to return, I felt the throb in my back. With increasing clarity came increasing pain. I was back in my reclining chair, locked into my brace, and suffering the pain of cancerous bones.

For a few hours, I had traded my pain for a drug induced journey to another space. It was not a trip I wanted to repeat. I was afraid I would lose my mind. I put aside the Levo Dromamine and resumed my Tylenol with codeine.

* * *

On the morning of October 15, I was admitted to the hospital for my first chemotherapy treatment. Ralph and my mother wheeled me around for the various preadmission procedures.

"You can get into bed," said the nurse who took us to my semi-private room.

"I can't," I told her. "I can't lie on a bed. I'll just sit here in the wheelchair."

"You need to be put on intravenous," she told me. "You'll be here overnight. You have to get into bed."

I told her that all my blood work had been done from my wheelchair, a cardiogram had been done from my wheelchair, and there was no reason why I couldn't have chemotherapy from my wheelchair. I explained that I was in pain, and sitting in a slouched semi-reclining position was more bearable than any bed.

She went to check with the head nurse. The head nurse came into my room and told me that I would have to get into the bed. She offered to help me.

Ralph adjusted the bed. He raised the back to a semi-reclining position, and he cranked up the bottom to support my legs. I popped some painkillers, and Ralph, my mother, and the two nurses helped me into the bed. I writhed in pain while Ralph adjusted the bed and maneuvered me until we found a bearable position. An intravenous was started.

To ensure that I would be fully hydrated for the chemo-therapy, an eighteen-hour flush had been prescribed. The intravenous would run all day, I would get the chemotherapy in the evening, and the intravenous would continue through the night. I would go home the next morning.

Ralph went to work, and my mother stayed with me all day. When Ralph came back, my mother went home to make din-ner for my father and Jeffrey. Ralph's dinner was a roll from a vending machine. I nibbled a little from my unappetizing hospital tray.

The CCNU consisted of two green pills. The Adriamycin was administered intravenously. For the first half hour noth-ing happened. Then a queasiness began in my stomach, followed by nausea. Heaving, gagging, choking, and then, "I'm going to throw up." Ralph looked around, grabbed the nearest wastebasket, and held it up to my face. The smell of the wastebasket made the nausea worse. I started vomiting, and when I thought I had finished, I started again.

Ralph rang for a nurse. As soon as she entered the room she started to laugh. It was a funny sight—me slouched over in the bed and Ralph bending over me with the wastebasket into which I gagged and vomited. The nurse opened my bedside table and took out a plastic dishpan. "Here," she said to Ralph, handing it to him and taking away the wastebasket. "We use this for vomiting."

All night I heaved and vomited. By morning I was ex-hausted, sapped of any energy that I might still have had. I felt drained, limp and listless, a spaghetti person.

"What did they do to you?" my mother asked when she and my father came to help Ralph take me out of the car and into the house.

"They poisoned me," I answered tearfully. "They pumped me full of poisons."

* * *

I drifted in and out of sleep. I was too weak to reach for
my painkillers. Someone put them in my mouth when I asked,
and in a notebook, my family jotted down the times when I
took each pill. The notebooks quickly filled up.

Ralph put a cot in the living room next to the reclining
chair, and my family took turns spending the night with me.
Whoever spent the night didn't get much sleep—every half
hour I needed another pill, or my position had to be changed
to relieve the pressure on my back.

My Dad was a heavy sleeper, and in his shift as night nurse
he was afraid that if he dozed off and I called him, he would
not hear me. He gave me a long stick, and I promised that I
would tap him with it if he fell asleep.

Every time he dozed off I tried desperately to bear the pain
so as not wake him, but I always had to resort to the stick.
He didn't mind; it was all he could do for me, and he wanted
to contribute in any way he could.

The pain was horrendous. I thought it couldn't possibly get
worse. Sometimes in the midst of a torturous, agonizing
spasm, I would beg Ralph to try to get me some cyanide. I
couldn't bear the pain.

I hated being such a heavy burden to my family. I didn't
want them to have to watch me disintegrate and suffer. I
didn't want to cause them this anguish. Maybe it would be
better if I died, I thought. Maybe it would be better to die
now, before I lost my mind as well as my body, before my
family would come to hope for my death as they now hoped
for my life.

I thought about writing a living will. If I reached the point
where there was no hope for my recovery from extreme physical or mental disability, I didn't want to be kept alive by
medication, artificial means, or other heroic efforts. I wanted
to die in peace. I didn't want my family to remember me as
a sick, degenerated, pain-riddled invalid to whom life had
become such a painful burden.

But I couldn't die now. Jeffrey was still a little boy. How could I die and leave him? And Rhonda was in Israel. How could I die and leave a daughter alone on the other side of the world? How could I leave Debra and Rachel in the midst of their growing accomplishments, in the midst of their youth? Who would love Ralph if I died now? How could I leave Ralph with no one to love? And my parents? How could I allow them to watch their oldest child suffer and die?

I was not afraid to die. Death would be a blessing now, a release from pain, a welcome peace. But I didn't want to die. I wasn't ready yet. I wasn't finished living.

* * *

My chemotherapy treatment was followed by five more radiation treatments, which were followed by another cycle of chemotherapy on November 23. Again I vomited all night. Again I felt nauseous for days, and weak, tired, and withered for weeks.

Gradually, the severity of my pain decreased and the spasms lessened in frequency and duration. The radiation had done what it was supposed to do. It reduced the sharp, piercing, burning torture to pain that was not so chronically unbearable.

Ralph rented a hospital bed. I couldn't lie on it. We tried a firmer mattress. I still couldn't lie on it. The back of the bed was adjustable but the front didn't elevate. I couldn't keep my legs straight; that was too painful. He returned the bed and ordered another. Both the back and the front of this bed could be adjusted, and the entire bed could be raised or lowered. I managed to get somewhat comfortable when I was positioned in this bed. We ordered a special buzzer, a walkie-talkie type of device. When I pushed a button by the bed, a loud buzzer went off in the kitchen. The buzzer sent someone running to my room.

I kept sliding down in the bed, and there was no way I could reposition myself. Two people were always needed to help me. Each grabbed one of my arms, I planted my feet firmly on the mattress, and we counted, "one, two, three, —now," and I closed my eyes and winced while they pulled me back into position Shortly afterwards I would begin to slide down again. When I slid down to the point where I was in tremendous pain, I rang the buzzer and help came. We repeated this process throughout the day and night.

I developed a twitching and tingling in my legs. Sometimes my legs would shake uncontrollably, sometimes they jumped into the air and fell down again. They twitched and trembled and rested by their own will; I could neither command them to move nor to stay still.

I stayed in the hospital bed with my pills and my buzzer. Ralph, Debra, and Rachel went to work, Jeffrey went to school, my Dad went home to Florida and came back again. Shayndee and Phyllis continued to come regularly, and their visits were the highlights of my days. My friends did the grocery shopping. They prepared soups, salads, and casseroles. They chauffered Jeffrey to wherever he needed to go— school events, parties, ice-skating, the movies. My mother never left the house. As long as I was confined to the bed, my mother wanted to be there.

One job was exclusively Ralph's. Every morning he injected me with vitamin B_{12} and Folic Acid. My oncologist had recommended that I come in to the hospital every day for the injections, a physical impossibility for me. We could find no nurse who would come to the house, and the daily injections were needed to offset, at least in part, the devastating effects that the chemotherapy was having on my blood. Ralph had spent a morning in the hospital practicing by injecting an orange. When he had mastered the technique, B_{12} Folic Acid, sterile gauze pads, alcohol, needles, and syringes took their place beside my painkillers. An assortment of laxatives completed our drugstore.

* * *

"How about a shower?" Ralph suggested.

"A shower!" I repeated. "How can I stand in the shower? How would I even get there?"

It was the morning of December 5. My parents, Debra, Rachel, and Jeffrey were spending the day with Phyllis and her family in the celebration of her son's Bar-Mitzvah. Ralph and I were alone.

Ralph had an idea. He would put our six-legged walker in the shower and adjust the water. Then he would carry me to the shower and support me while I held on to the walker.

"I can't do that," I told him.

"Let's try," he said. "You can hold on to the walker and lean against me. It'll just take a few minutes."

We both knew that I needed a shower desperately. I had been using a bedpan first on the recliner and then on the hospital bed, and very often I would get my clothes wet. We kept waterproof pads on the bed, and my nightgown was changed regularly, but we didn't change the tee shirt under my brace. Removing the brace, removing the tee shirt and getting me into another one was too painful and traumatic for me. I would rather smell than endure the pain. Ralph was embarrassed when anyone came into the room and when we went to the hospital for my treatments. The odor had become offensive.

"I'll try," I said. "But I don't want you to carry me. I'll try to walk holding on to you and the walker."

We shuffled a few steps towards the bathroom.

"Can you hold on to the walker for a minute while I check the water?" Ralph asked.

"Sure," I said.

Ralph adjusted the water. I turned my head slightly and looked in the mirror. What I saw horrified me.

My head was completely bald. My face was pale, the bones in my neck stuck out, and my abdomen was so distended that I looked very pregnant. My thighs and my buttocks were completely black and blue from my daily injections, and black and blue splotches dotted my arms and legs. My back was all marked up with purple and red lines, x's, and other assorted markings from my radiation treatments. My back muscles had atrophied from disuse and my backbone jutted out—a purple and black protrusion that ended at my lower spine in a mass of red and purple and black broken bone.

"Ralph!" I screamed.

Ralph caught me as I fainted, just as I was about to hit the floor.

I suffered agonizing back pain, a twisted ankle, and a bent toe that immediately turned black and blue. Ralph carried me back to bed, and I slept away most of the day.

I woke up feeling angry. Angry at what had become of me. How could anyone stand to look at me? It was not human to look like that, to smell like that, to feel like that. I was filled with revulsion and disgust. And anger.

I pressed my buzzer and Ralph came running.

"I'm okay now," I told him. "I'll take my shower now."

Ralph thought it would be better to wait for another time. But I was determined. "Please help me," I pleaded. "I want a shower so badly. I'm sure I can do it now."

This time Ralph did not let go of me. We shuffled over to the shower, and Ralph held me in one arm as he adjusted the water with the other. Then we showered together—Ralph, me, and the walker.

It was my first shower in four months.

* * *

My father had not been feeling well. He did not sleep well at night, he felt weak and tired during the day, he looked pale, and he lacked energy. On December 23, after our annual family Chanukah party, my parents went back to Florida.

Because I could not be transported, the Chanukah party was held at my house. Store-bought potato pancakes with applesauce, traditional Chanukah food, replaced the usual

full-course festive meal. I stayed upstairs in my hospital
bed until it was time for candle lighting and gift giving. Then
I joined my family in the living room where I sat in my
recliner, grateful that I had survived another Chanukah, hoping that this would not be my last.

On December 28, my Dad was admitted to the hospital
with severe anemia. Even after his release, he was not well
enough to come back to New Jersey. My mother was torn;
she wanted to take care of him and she wanted to take care
of me. We assured my parents that we could manage, and
we all agreed that they should stay in Florida until Jeffrey's
Bar-Mitzvah, which would be at the end of February.

When we had learned of the metastasis of my cancer in
October, Ralph cancelled the plans we had made for Jeffrey's
Bar-Mitzvah. I had been upset; I hadn't wanted to deprive
my son of a Bar-Mitzvah celebration. But Ralph had insisted
that he would not have a celebration without me. How could
he give a party while I was suffering such pain? How could
he plan a celebration when neither of us knew if I would still
be alive when the time came?

With the reduction of my pain from the radiation, we had
reinstated our plans. I would come to the service in my wheelchair, and I would stay until I got tired. Rhonda would come
home from Israel, and our family and our friends would join
us in celebration.

My third cycle of chemotherapy was administered on
December 17, and my fourth was on January 7, 1983. On
January 8 I had chest X-rays, and on January 18, I had spinal
X-rays and a bone scan.

Ralph was planning a business trip to Europe on January
22. A week of appointments had been arranged in England,
France, and Germany. He planned to leave on Saturday night,
January 22 and return home on Sunday, January 31.

Rachel had a few days vacation time, and she planned to
take them while Ralph was away. When her vacation days
were used up, she and Debra would take care of me in the

morning before leaving for work, and again in the evenings. Friends would pitch in during the day. We thought we would be able to manage.

* * *

Tuesday, January 18

We returned from the hospital after my spinal X-rays and bone scan. Ralph put me to bed, and before leaving for work, he brought up the mail.

I opened an envelope and felt a sharp pain run across my left hand. Blood oozed from between my thumb and my index finger. I wiped up the blood and saw that I had a paper-cut.

Wednesday, January 19

My hand throbbed. The area around the paper-cut looked red and puffy.

"Better call the doctor," Ralph said.

"Which doctor?" I asked him.

"The oncologist," he answered.

"The oncologist!" I repeated. "I can't bother the oncologist with a little paper-cut."

"Call the family doctor then," Ralph persisted. "Maybe he'll prescribe some antibiotics."

"I don't know if I can take antibiotics while I'm on chemotherapy," I said.

"You've got to do something," Ralph insisted.

"I will," I promised. "If it doesn't feel better this afternoon, I'll call the oncologist."

By afternoon my hand was purple and swollen.

Thursday, January 20

I reached my oncologist and described the paper-cut.

"Put Bacitracin ointment on every few hours," she told me. "Call me back if it doesn't get better."

I didn't have any Bacitracin.

I called my friend Evelyn. No answer. I called some
other friends. No one was home. Finally I reached Felice.
Felice went to the drugstore to get the Bacitracin.

"I don't like the way that looks," Felice said when she
saw my hand.

"Don't worry," I assured her. "It's just a little paper-
cut."

By evening my whole hand felt numb. The swelling had
traveled to my wrist.

Friday, January 21

I called the doctor again.

"Come right in," she said. "I want to take a look at it."

I couldn't come right in. I was lying in my hospital bed,
in my brace, barely able to move. How could I come right
in?

I didn't want to bother Ralph at work. Tomorrow night
he would be leaving for Europe. He had a lot of last minute things to take care of, and I knew he was very busy.
But who else could dress me, help me down the stairs,
drive me to the hospital, and get me from the car into a
wheelchair?

I called the doctor back and reached her nurse.

"How late will the doctor be in today?" I asked her.

"Until four o'clock," she said. "Be sure to be here before
four."

Ralph came home at three-thirty. He dressed me in my
sweat suit. I wore sweat pants and an extra large sweat
shirt each time we went to the hospital. It was the only
thing that fit over my bulky brace. Ralph had done some
shopping on his way home. Before we left for the hospital,
he put two chickens in the oven, one for the weekend and
one to freeze for when he would be away. He wrote a note
for Jeffrey, who would be coming home from school soon. "I
took Mommy to the hospital to show the doctor her paper-
cut," the note said. "We'll be home in a little while."

"Let me see your hand," my oncologist said to me as she walked into her office.

I raised my hand slightly.

She picked up the phone. "Admitting," I heard her say. "I need a bed immediately."

*　*　*

I did not think the doctor was talking about me. She had taken a quick glance at my hand, and I thought that now she was taking care of someone else before getting back to me.

"N-U-S-S-B-A-U-M," she was spelling into the phone.

I snapped to attention.

"Me?" I questioned her from my wheelchair. "Are you admitting me?"

She nodded.

"Why?" I asked. "I just came to show you my paper-cut."

She was talking into the phone again. She said something about a massive infection. She wasn't sure if it had penetrated the bone. She wanted a plastic surgeon to look at it tonight. No, it couldn't wait until tomorrow, it had to be tonight.

She dialed another number. She was sending a patient up right now, she said. She gave my name. She wanted an intravenous started immediately. I would need massive doses of intravenous antibiotics.

I just stared at her, dumbfounded. "Wait a minute," I said when I found my voice. "You can't admit me now. I have to go home now."

She would not allow me to leave. I had a massive infection, cellulitis of the finger, the hand, and the arm. There weren't enough white corpuscles in my body to fight infection. Untreated, I could die from the paper-cut.

Debra was in New York for the weekend. Rachel was in Florida visiting my parents. Rhonda was in Israel. Jeffrey was home alone with the two chickens in the oven. And Ralph was leaving tomorrow night for a week-long trip to Europe.

"I didn't bring a nightgown," I said to the oncologist. "Or a toothbrush. I didn't make any arrangements at home. Suppose I go home now and check in tomorrow morning."

She insisted that I not leave the hospital. Ralph could go home and pack a bag for me. I needed to start heavy anti-biotic treatment immediately.

"Why can't I take antibiotics orally?" I persisted. I really didn't want to stay in the hospital.

I would need massive doses of antibiotics intravenously to ensure immediate infusion into my blood stream. I would also need blood transfusions—my red cells, white cells, and plate-lets were all dangerously low. And she wanted a surgeon to look at my hand.

"How long will I be in the hospital?" I asked.

She could not project. She knew only that it would be a few days at least.

We called Debra in New York. No answer. We called Rachel in Florida. She would come before Ralph left for Europe. We called Shayndee. No answer. We called Phyllis. She would come and bring Jeffrey home with her.

At five o'clock, January 21, 1983, I was admitted to the hospital with uterine cancer that had spread to my bones and my lungs, deep tendonitis of my finger, hand, and arm, and a grossly suppressed immune system.

* * *

The plastic surgeon examined my hand while his assistant looked on. "We'll have to cut all around here," he said, pointing to the area around my paper-cut. "I think we'll be able to save the hand."

On Saturday morning, the surgeon, his assistant, and two nurses arrived at my bedside with a cart full of instruments and assorted bandages. One of the nurses suggested that I look the other way, which I did, and I tried not to scream while surgery was performed on my left hand.

I was bandaged from my wrist to the tips of my fingers. Rolls of gauze were wrapped around my wound. My hand looked like it was wearing an oversized white boxing glove. My treatment would consist of warm moist heat applied locally to my hand, elevation of my arm, and antibiotic treatment with Nafcillin and Flagil.

A tank of water and a water heater were brought to my left side. Water passed through the heater and then through the rubber tubing that ran from the heater to my bandaged hand. My arm was placed on a pile of three pillows, the top of which was covered with waterproof padding. The water flowed constantly, my hand remained drenched, and excess water continued to dribble up my arm no matter how often the nurses rearranged the pillows.

On my other side stood the intravenous apparatus, from which antibiotics dripped steadily into a vein in my right arm. Another intravenous pole held bags of washed blood. The washed blood passed through a blood warmer before being transfused into my body. The blood warmer stood on a table next to the intravenous poles.

I lay between the water tank, the water heater, and the pillows on one side, and the blood, the bloodwarmer, and the intravenous poles on the other side. A scarf covered my bald head, a brace encased my aching body, rubber tubes ran into both my bandaged arms. A pitiful sight. The result of a paper-cut.

* * *

I was nervous about Ralph being in Europe while I was in the hospital. He had been at my side throughout every procedure, and I had come to depend on his being there. I knew that he could be home within an hour if ever I needed him while he was working. Now he was going to Europe and leaving me alone in the hospital. I felt abandoned. And I was scared.

"Don't go," I begged him. "Cancel the trip."

The trip couldn't be cancelled. Everything was already arranged and confirmed.

"Send someone else," I pleaded.

There was no one who could leave for Europe at a moment's notice and implement any sort of a plan.

"I'm scared," I told Ralph. "I'm scared to be here in the hospital when you're so far away."

Ralph was in a quandry. He wanted to do right by me and he wanted to do right by his job. This was to be his first visit to Europe, a necessary trip to get involved in the European aspect of his responsibilities. He wanted to keep his job. He needed to keep his job. What could he do for me while I was in the hospital? I was just lying there, all bandaged up, getting antibiotics and blood transfusions. A doctor would see me every day, Ralph assured me, and the nurses would take care of me.

I didn't want doctors and nurses. I wanted Ralph.

Ralph talked it over with the children. This might be only one incident of many, they agreed. Ralph had to keep his job. He would go through with the trip to Europe.

* * *

Despite four blood transfusions and massive doses of intravenous antibiotics, my white blood count remained critically low. I was put in reverse isolation.

Reverse isolation, I learned, differed from regular isolation in its purpose. The purpose of isolation is to isolate the patient so that he cannot communicate his illness to others. Reverse isolation isolates the patient for his own protection, against any germs, infections, or illnesses that others may have or be harboring. No one with a cold, a cough, a sore throat, an infection, an open wound, or an illness of any kind, was allowed to come near me.

On the door to my room, which was kept closed at all times, was posted a sign, "ISOLATION ROOM." Next to the door stood a table which held paper robes, paper hats, paper face masks, and rubber gloves. Anyone entering my room, including the doctors and nurses, had to first dress himself in this outfit.

Debra had a cold. She could not visit or help me in any way. Sole responsibility fell onto Rachel.

On January 24, another set of X-rays were taken of my lungs and my spine. The X-rays were scheduled in the evening so that Rachel could be there to help me with my brace.

Rachel and I were dressed up in sterile isolation costumes. My intravenous pole was attached to my wheelchair, and I was ordered to keep my left hand raised throughout the entire procedure. "We're bringing her down now," the nurse notified the X-ray department. Anyone not necessary for the procedure was asked to leave the department. There were to be no extra people milling around. Anyone with a cold was ordered to leave the area immediately. All technicians were told to be dressed in sterile gowns and masks.

A nurse preceded us to make sure that no one would breathe on me in the corridors or in the elevator. Rachel wheeled me into the X-ray room, unfastened my brace, and helped me onto the X-ray table. When the X-rays were finished, she refastened my brace, wheeled me back to my room and helped me back into bed.

"Did you tell the doctor about your stomach?" Rachel asked me.

"What about my stomach?" I answered.

"It's tremendous," Rachel said. "You look like you're about to give birth."

I reminded Rachel that my swollen belly was from all the medication and the fluids I was getting. Nothing to worry about. Rachel insisted that I have someone look at it.

The next morning, four interns and residents came in to look at my stomach. They poked and palpated, and they agreed that the abnormal distention was due to fluid effusion into my abdominal cavity. "If it doesn't go down in a few days," one of them said, "we'll have to puncture and drain it."

The swelling didn't go down, and no one remembered to check it again. I didn't remind them. The thought of having my stomach punctured and drained did not particularly appeal to me.

Rachel came to the hospital early every morning and fed me breakfast before leaving for work. She came back in time to help me with supper, and she stayed until she was ordered to leave.

My friends Evelyn, Evelyn, and Eunice came almost every day, bearing food, flowers, and magazines. The first time their visits overlapped, they didn't recognize each other. In their isolation costumes, with only their eyes showing, everyone looked alike. They took turns feeding me lunch and trying to cheer me up.

Ralph's brother, Jack, came often in the evenings. Jack brought snacks, magazines, and one night he arrived with a tiny portable radio that fit on the side of my bed. Shayndee and Phyllis came on alternating nights, and sometimes we shared a picnic dinner on my bed. "Do you still like the dark meat?" Shayndee asked one evening when she arrived with barbecued chicken, sweet potatoes. And cole slaw.

"I sure do," I told her. "And I love sweet potatoes."

"Me too," said Shayndee.

All the nurses agreed that for someone who didn't have full use of her hands, I was eating better than anyone else on the floor.

Every morning and evening, vials of blood were drawn from my arm for analysis. Every morning my bandages were changed, and sometimes this procedure included some cutting away of my skin. My hand had become white and shriveled, it throbbed constantly, it itched, and it felt slimy. I had an overwhelming urge to rip off the bandages, wrap my poor wet shriveled hand in a warm dry towel, and nurse it back to health.

Towards the end of the week, the water dripping into my hand was discontinued, and the antibiotics were gradually reduced as my white blood count began to slowly increase. I was released from the hospital on Sunday, January 30, the same day that Ralph returned from Europe.

My intake of Megace was increased to eight hundred milligrams daily, to be taken three times a day in the form of twenty tablets. I was given a prescription for two kinds of oral antibiotics. I was to continue to take my vitamins. I would be swallowing thirty-eight pills a day.

I was told that I would not be able to complete my initial protocol of chemotherapy. It was too toxic for my blood; it could destroy me before the cancer would. I would be put on something milder.

My new treatment would consist of two hundred milligrams of Cytoxan, given intravenously, once every month. I was to begin on February 16.

* * *

My bone scan on July 28, 1982 showed a compression fracture.

My X-rays and bone scan on September 28 showed cancer on my lower spine and a mass on my lung.

My chest X-rays on January 8, 1983 showed no change in my lungs, and my bone scan on January 18 showed no change in my bones.

My X-rays on January 24 showed a "shadow" on my upper back.

That's what I had been told.

* * *

Apparently, my doctors had felt that it would be better if I did not know the severity of my condition. It was only later, when I requested my medical records that I learned the true extent of my illness. It read as follows:

July 28, 1982—Compression fracture of L2. [lower spine]
September 28, 1982—Metastatic disease to L2. [cancer on
lower spine]
Metastatic disease to T9. [cancer on
middle spine]
Multiple metastatic deposits in both
lungs. [cancerous nodules of differ-
ent sizes in both lungs]
January 8, 1983—Metastatic lung disease—unchanged.
January 18, 1983—Increased activity in L2.
Increase in degree of compression of L2.
Increased activity in T9.
Destruction and partial compression of
T9.
Progression of metastatic disease in T9.
[cancer spreading]
January 24, 1983—Complete collapse of L2.
Progressive metastatic disease to L2 and
T9. [cancer spreading]
Bilateral pulmonary nodules consistent
with metastatic disease. [cancer
spreading in both lungs]

* * *

Two hundred milligrams of Cytoxan a month! Twice I had
taken four hundred milligrams for five consecutive days. For
eight months I had taken one hundred fifty milligrams a day
orally. I had taken Adriamycin and CCNU which proved too
toxic for my blood. I had undergone radical surgery. I had
received megadoses of radiation. I had endured a seventy-two
hour radium implant. Nothing had succeeded in stopping the
advancing cancer. What could I expect now from two hundred milligrams of Cytoxan a month?

"Why?" I wondered. Why was this happening to me? I

was a good person, as good as most people and better than some who were walking around in the best of health. My doctors had given me the best medical care, and I had followed their instructions implicitly, doing exactly what I was told to do. I had prayed so much, my family and my friends had prayed, we had begged and pleaded for my life. Where was God? Why wasn't He listening? Where was mercy? Where was justice?

Part II

Two roads diverged in a wood,
and I—I took the one less traveled by,
And that has made all the difference."

—ROBERT FROST

Chapter 5

THE ARTICLE HAD APPEARED IN A PHILADELPHIA NEWSPAPER. It told about a medical doctor who had freed himself of terminal cancer with a macrobiotic diet. The article, dated January 9, 1983, stated that the doctor had written a book about his tortured journey to the edge of death and his return to vigorous life. I had decided to save the article.

"What do you know about a macrobiotic diet?" I asked my friend Evelyn Ash as she and Rachel sat by my hospital bed during my paper cut treatments.

Evelyn knew nothing about it. I told her about the article.

"You ought to try it," Evelyn suggested.

"The doctor saw someone in Philadelphia," I said. "I don't know if there's anyone in New York or New Jersey."

"I'll drive you to Philadelphia," Evelyn volunteered.

"It's a long way to Philadelphia," I said. "I wouldn't ask you to take me there. Suppose I would have to go back regularly?"

"You didn't ask me," Evelyn said. "I offered. If you want to do it, I'll take you there as often as you need to go."

"I can take you sometimes, too," Rachel said. "We can stay overnight so you won't have to sit in the car all day. We can work it out."

"Do you remember the name of the book the doctor wrote?" I asked Rachel.

She didn't remember, and neither did I. I told her where to find the newspaper article.

The next morning, before she left the hospital for work, Rachel gave me a slip of paper. On it was written, "*Recalled by Life*, by Dr. Anthony Sattilaro."

I gave the paper to Evelyn. "Try the library," I told her. "If they don't have it, try Barnes and Noble, and if they don't have it, maybe Rachel can get it in New York."

"I'll get it," Evelyn promised. And she did.

I read the book. I read certain segments again. This man had been riddled with cancer. Despite the fact that he was a doctor, that he had access to the best medical care, his professional colleagues could offer him no hope, and he had resigned himself to a short and painful future. Then he discovered macrobiotics. Within six weeks his pain disappeared, within a few months the course of his illness was reversed, and after fifteen months of macrobiotic eating, his bone scan showed no cancer cells.

I thought about macrobiotics. "It's just food," I told myself. Unlike many other alternative treatments, there was nothing expensive, difficult, or unpleasant about it. I would not have to travel to Germany, Sweden, or Tiajuana. I would not need to take injections, pills, or colonics. I would not need to squeeze thirteen glasses of carrot juice every day, eat only wheat grass, or only raw foods. I would need only to eat balanced meals. My knowledge of macrobiotics was very limited, but based on what I already knew, this diet made sense.

One thought kept recurring. The doctor had been riddled with cancer, and now he was well. "If he could do it," I said to myself, "Why can't I?"

I decided to investigate macrobiotics. It was the first week in February.

* * *

I maneuvered my wheelchair to the telephone and called information. I dialed the number that the operator gave me.

"I'm a cancer patient and I'm interested in macrobiotics," I told the person on the other end. "Could you send me some information?"

"Would you like to come in and see someone?" he asked me.

"I can't," I answered. "I'm in a wheelchair and a brace, and there's no way I can make the trip to New York. Could you send me some literature so that I can get started on my own?"

"Where do you live?" he asked.

"In West Orange, New Jersey," I told him.

"There's someone in New Jersey who might be able to help you," he said. And he gave me the number of Arthur Jackson.

Arthur Jackson had developed prostate trouble more than twenty years ago, and his doctors had told him that his prostate would have to be removed. He had also suffered from rheumatoid arthritis. His joints had been damaged from years of taking medications, he had worn specially molded shoes that enabled him to walk—he had been almost crippled. In his search for a method of natural healing, he had attended a seminar at the United Nations that was hosted by Gloria Swanson and Bill Dufty. It was there that he had been introduced to macrobiotics.

He had begun eating macrobiotically, and he had started feeling better. His arthritic pain had decreased, his prostate had gradually improved, and his hair had become thicker and darker. Now, at the age of seventy-one, he had outlived his two urologists and was enjoying good health. He was a firm believer in macrobiotics, and he was very willing to give of himself and to help others.

"I'll send you a copy of the standard macrobiotic diet," Arthur said after I told him my own story. "Read it over, discuss it with your husband, and if you're interested, call me back and we'll talk some more."

I studied the papers that Arthur sent me. The basic macrobiotic diet, I learned, consisted of fifty to sixty percent whole grains, twenty-five to thirty percent locally grown vegetables, about ten percent beans and sea vegetables, and five percent soups. Various seasonings, condiments, and beverages were included, as were supplemental foods such as fish, fruit, and nuts and seeds. Foods to be avoided included all meat, poultry, eggs, dairy food, simple sugars, chemicalized foods, refined grains and flours, canned and frozen foods, tropical fruits and juices, and vitamin supplements. The papers also included a list of "way of life suggestions" that seemed easy enough to follow.

"I'm going to do this," I decided, even before I showed the papers to Ralph and the children. "I'm definitely going to do this."

The whole grains will be no problem, I thought to myself. I loved hot cereal. And I loved vegetables. Some of my favorite vegetables, like asparagus and sweet potatoes, were to be avoided, but there was a large enough variety from the permissible vegetables to choose from. Beans would be no problem and neither would soups, but I wasn't sure about the sea vegetables. I had never heard of *wakame, kombu, arame,* or *hijiki;* I couldn't even pronounce the words. Where would I buy them? How would I prepare them? Maybe I could just skip that part of the diet. I would ask Arthur.

I made a list of questions. "I can't cook very much from my wheelchair," I told Arthur. "Can my husband cook the food on Sunday for the whole week? Can I just leave out the foods I don't like? Can I skip the sea vegetables altogether? What's *miso?* Where will I get calcium and vitamin C if I don't eat dairy food and fruit? What's wrong with vitamin pills? Can I do this myself, or do I have to see a advisor?"

Arthur told me that I should see a advisor as soon as I possibly could. He also recommended that I take cooking lessons. He said it was perfectly okay for me to call him whenever I had any questions.

I had a multitude of questions. I kept a running list and I called Arthur every few days. He always had time and patience for me.

Jeffrey's Bar-Mitzvah was on Sunday, February 27, on the holiday of Purim. I came to the Synagogue in my wheelchair, a maternity dress to cover my bulky brace, and a wig to cover my still bald head. I ate nothing from the festive buffet lunch that was served; I ate only the rice and vegetables that I brought along. It was a beautiful Bar-Mitzvah. Jeffrey's performance was outstanding, and we were all very proud of him.

For the first time in a long while, I felt good about myself. Finally, I was doing something positive. I felt in control; through my diet I could control my body. "It's going to work," I told myself over and over. "This diet is going to work for me. It has to. It's my only hope."

* * *

I ate grains and vegetables almost exclusively. Every few days, Ralph cooked a pot of rice and cut up some vegetables for me. I was able to maneuver my wheelchair to the refrigerator, take out the food, warm up the rice, and boil or steam the vegetables. We kept two pots on the stove at all times so I didn't have to reach or bend. A typical meal consisted of rice and some vegetables such as squash, kale, carrots, or broccoli. I was satisfied.

On March 7, Arthur Jackson came to see me. He brought a folder full of reading material, a few copies of the *East West Journal* magazine, and a book called *The Macrobiotic Approach to Cancer* by Michio Kushi. For two hours we talked about macrobiotics.

"What did you plan for lunch today?" Arthur asked me.

"Rice and vegetables," I told him. "Would you like to join me?"

"I'd love to," Arthur said. "I'll cook lunch for us."

Out of my refrigerator came an assortment of vegetables. I told Arthur where to find a big pot and a knife.

"We'll have stoup," Arthur announced.

"What's stoup?" I asked him. I didn't remember reading anything about stoup.

"It's a combination of stew and soup," Arthur explained. "I made up the word myself."

Arthur cut and cooked the vegetables. He added some cooked rice and seasoned the dish with tamari soy sauce. It was delicious, by far the best lunch I had had in a long time.

Arthur suggested that I take macrobiotic cooking lessons as soon as I was able to get around a little. He told me that a woman named Hilda Sorhagen was teaching macrobiotic cooking in Whippany, which was only about a twenty minute drive from West Orange.

Evelyn Ash had also told me about Hilda. Evelyn had been in the beauty parlor where she heard two women talking about macrobiotics. One of the women told Evelyn that she had taken cooking lessons with Hilda. Evelyn had offered to drive me there whenever I was ready to go.

I called Hilda. Hilda herself had had cancer. She had healed herself with macrobiotics and was opening up her home to teach macrobiotic cooking to others. She was starting a new series of classes the next night, March 8. They would run for six consecutive Tuesdays, from seven o'clock until nine or nine-thirty. She suggested that Ralph and I take the classes.

"I can't come at night," I told her. "Is there anything available during the day?"

There wasn't. "Why can't you come in the evening?" Hilda asked me.

I told her about my condition and explained that I get very tired at night. I couldn't always stay up until nine o'clock. I also told her that Ralph traveled quite a bit and he would not always be available to take me.

"What about private or semi-private lessons during the day?" I asked Hilda. I offered to pay for any additional expense.

Hilda couldn't accommodate me in the daytime. She also

felt that it was important for Ralph to take the lessons too. "Who will cook for you if you get sick?" she asked me.

Ralph and I talked it over. "It's up to you," he said. "If you think you're up to it, I'll take you at night."

I was not up to it physically. But I didn't want to wait until the next series which would be two months away at the earliest. Based on my reading, I knew that cooking classes were important, and I wanted to take them.

"Let's try," I said to Ralph. "I'll take a long nap in the late afternoon, and if I get tired at the class, we can just leave early."

Every Tuesday night, from March 8 until April 12, Ralph and I studied macrobiotic cooking. Our class included another couple—the wife had breast cancer, a young woman who was learning to cook for her husband who had liver cancer and was too weak to come to class, several other cancer patients, and a few people with other degenerative diseases. We all sat around Hilda's kitchen table and took notes. That is, everyone else sat around the table. I stood. Every week I hobbled in on Ralph's arm with my walker or with a cane. In my sweat pants, bulky sweater, sneakers, and scarf, I leaned against the wall or held on to a chair and listened, watched, and asked a lot of questions.

Hilda was assisted by Karen Davis, a young, slim woman with a peaches-and-cream complexion. Karen had a light and airy quality about her, and she added a refreshing touch to the class. Together they cooked soups, grains, vegetables, and beans. I liked the food, and some of the dishes were really delicious. But not the sea vegetables. The *wakame* and *kombu* sea vegetables, which were cooked into the food, were tolerable, but the *arame* and *hijiki* side dishes tasted awful. Even the smell was offensive. In one class we made a condiment with *nori* sea vegetable, and I left the whole dish untouched. I liked the grains and the well-cooked vegetables best, Ralph liked the pressed salads, and we both loved the soups. Ralph bought me a new recipe box, I copied my notes onto index cards, and I attempted to recreate at home what I had learned in class. I continued to restrict myself to grains, some beans, and vegetables.

* * *

I wanted to see Michio Kushi. From my readings and from talking to people, I learned that he was the highest authority on macrobiotics. I had heard that by a visual examination, by looking at a person's face, eyes, hands, arms, and sometimes his feet, Mr. Kushi could evaluate a person's condition and could recommend adjustments in the standard macrobiotic diet to the individual's specific needs. I felt certain that Michio Kushi could tell me if macrobiotics would work for me if I would follow his advice exactly.

Arthur Jackson gave me the number of the East West Foundation in Brookline, Massachusetts, where Michio Kushi taught. I called to arrange for a visit.

The waiting list to talk with Mr. Kushi was four months long. The person on the phone offered to add my name to the list and to call me back in three months to arrange a definite meeting.

I felt instant disappointment and fear. I knew I couldn't wait four months.

"I'm a cancer patient," I said to the person on the phone, "and I'm newly macrobiotic. Do you think I should wait for Mr. Kushi, or should I see someone else?"

"You should see someone soon," I was told. "We have a lot of qualified instructors right here in Brookline."

"I live in New Jersey," I said. "Is there anyone I can see in the New York-New Jersey area?"

"Oh yes," she answered enthusiastically. "If you can get to New York, see Shizuko Yamamoto. She's the best person to see."

I had read about Shizuko Yamamoto. I had also heard about her from my aunt, my mother's sister who lived in Florida. My aunt was interested in macrobiotics, and she had sent me a large packet of information. "The best person to see is Michio Kushi," she had written in her accompanying letter, "but if you can't make the trip to Brookline, there's a woman in New York, Shizuko Yamamoto, who is second in command and excellent."

Now the Foundation was recommending this same person.

"Could you spell that for me?" I asked the person on the other end of the phone.

I marked down Shizuko Yamamoto's name and number, expressed my thanks, hung up and immediately dialed New York.

Shizuko Yamamoto answered the phone. She was very busy now, she told me, but she could arrange a meeting with me in three months. I felt devastated.

"Could you possibly see me sooner?" I begged. "I have cancer in my spine and my lungs. I'm in a wheelchair and a brace, I'm just starting macrobiotics, and I need a lot of help. Could you squeeze me in soon, please?"

"Can you come tomorrow morning at ten o'clock?" she asked me, "I have a cancellation and I can see you then."

My spritis soared.

"I think so," I told her. "I just have to check with my husband to make sure he can drive me. Hold the time, and I'll call you right back."

I dialed Ralph. "Ralph!" I said excitedly. "Can you take me to see Shizuko Yamamoto tomorrow morning at ten o'clock? Please say yes!"

"I have an important meeting tomorrow at ten," Ralph said. "What about one day next week?"

"Oh Ralph," I cried. Breifly I told him about my call to Michio Kushi's office and then to Shizuko Yamamoto. "What should we do?" I asked him "How can I give up this meeting?"

"You can't," Ralph said. "I'll work something out here and I'll take you."

"Thank you, thank you, thank you," I repeated happily. "I'll call her right now and tell her we'll be there."

* * *

In everyone's life, certain experiences are remembered because they were so happy, so sad, so painful, so exciting, or just so unusual. The first hour I spent with Shizuko Yamamoto on March 10, 1983 was all of these things—and more. It was the strangest happening I had ever experienced.

Shizuko answered the door. She was a middle aged woman, short, sturdily built, simply dressed, and barefoot. "Come in," she invited us in her Japanese accent. She asked us to remove our shoes and to wait a few minutes. She said she would be with us shortly.

Over the coat rack was a sign, "Please Remove Shoes," and under the coat rack several pairs of shoes were lined up.

"Why do we have to take our shoes off?" I asked Ralph.

"I don't know," he answered. "Maybe because they always take their shoes off in Japan."

Ralph took off his shoes and my sneakers and arranged them next to the others. He sat down and looked through some *East West Journal* magazines, and I leaned against a wall and held on to my walker.

A couple came out of an adjacent room and put on their shoes. Shizuko Yamamoto beckoned us in.

It was a large square room. In the center, on the floor, was a large mat covered with a thin blanket. Against one wall was a bookcase stacked with macrobiotic books and magazines, and by the front window stood a desk and a few chairs. Shizuko produced an index card, on which she wrote my name, address, phone number, the nature of my illness (cancer), and who recommended me (East West Foundation in Brookline). That was the extent of my medical history.

She studied my face for a few seconds and told me that I had eaten a lot of dairy food in the past. I admitted that I used to eat yogurt and cottage cheese every day, and that I had used a lot of hard cheese and milk. She said something about the poor condition of my kidneys. How could she know about my kidneys by looking at my face, I wondered.

As far as I knew, there was nothing wrong with my kidneys. Certainly, in all my medical examinations and tests, no doctor had ever even mentioned my kidneys. True, I was urinating very frequently, sometimes as often as every half hour, and the urge would come on so suddenly and with such intensity that I didn't always make it to the bathroom. I woke up on the average of twelve to fourteen times a night, and I always wore a sanitary napkin. I had discussed this problem of incontinence with every doctor and every intern and resident that I had had any contact with. One had suggested that I see a urologist. One had offered to prescribe pills that would stretch my bladder. One had recommended that I not drink between dinner and bedtime. The general consensus had been that the frequency and intensity was a result of the heavy radiation I had received. There was no solution for the condition—I would just have to live with it.

Now I told Shizuko Yamamoto about this problem. "Don't worry," she said unhesitantly. "Condition can improve."

Shizuko asked me to undress in the bathroom and to put on a robe. "Should I take off my brace?" I asked her. Everything except my underwear was to be removed, she told me, including my watch and my wedding band.

Ralph undressed me and removed my brace. He helped me into a robe, and when we were ready, I was asked to lie down on the mat on the floor. I just stood there, holding on to Ralph. "I can't get down," I told Shizuko. She and Ralph gently lowered me onto the mat, and Ralph pulled up a chair to watch what would happen next.

Shizuko probed every part of my body. She pressed and she rubbed and she tapped and she kneaded and she shook. She pushed and she pulled and she stretched and she pounded. She turned me onto my stomach and repeated the procedure on my back.

Ralph kept jumping out of his chair. "She has a bad back!" he tried to interrupt her. "That's where the tumor is!" he practically screamed. Shizuko paid no attention. She continued working on me.

Then the strangest thing happened. Shizuko pulled up a
chair and placed it next to me. Holding on to the back of the
chair, she stepped onto my buttocks and proceeded to walk
up and down my back. I moaned and groaned and sometimes
I screamed when she stepped on certain spots. Ralph was
nearly hysterical. He sat rigidly on the edge of his chair, ready
to pounce, and I thought he was going to grab this woman
off me and toss her out the window. She ignored him, and
when she finished stomping on my back, she walked up and
down the backs of my legs, and then she stood on the soles
of my feet. I screamed. "I know, I know," she answered my
screams. "Kidneys too tight."

She helped me roll over onto my back again. She took my
pulse—my pulses—six of them. She sat down on her knees
alongside of me and she pressed certain spots on my body
while telling me, "breathe in, breathe out, breathe in, breathe
out." I breathed along with her, and I could feel my body
vibrating beneath her touch. I felt as if the pain was being
drawn out of me, and a warmth, a peacefulness was seeping
in. I looked up at Shizuko. She was kneeling beside me, her
eyes were closed, and she was rhythmically raising and lower-
ing her hands over various parts of my body while chanting,
"breathe in, breathe out." I closed my eyes too, and we
breathed together. I felt a sense of well-being, of content-
ment, of peacefulness.

Thus, I was introduced to *shiatsu* massage.

* * *

Shiatsu is an Oriental massage in which the fingers are
pressed on particular points of the body to ease tension,
fatigue, aches, pains, and symptoms of disease. *Shiatsu* helps
to maintain health, to strengthen energy, vitality, and stamina
in the body.

Barefoot *shiatsu* involves the use of the feet, which can be
as sensitive as the hand. Using the feet allows the practi-

tioner to keep his posture straight, enabling him to breathe more deeply and give a deeper, fuller *shiatsu* without becoming tired. The *shiatsu* practitioner must be strong and healthy, must have clear and precise thinking, and must have high intelligence and well-developed intuition.

Shizuko Yamamoto was an acknowledged master of the art of *shiatsu* in America, Europe, and Japan.

After my *shiatsu* was finished and I was dressed again, Shizuko gave me a macrobiotic food list, and we discussed my dietary recommendations. My diet would consist of sixty percent whole grains, about twenty-five percent vegetables, some beans and sea vegetables, and one or two bowls of *miso* soup daily. My primary grain would be pressure-cooked brown rice, and my secondary grains would be millet and barley. I was to avoid buckwheat and buckwheat noodles, and I was not to mix more than two grains in the same dish. I was to have one cup of *miso* soup each morning, prepared with vegetables and *wakame* sea vegetable. This soup would have to be prepared fresh every day. Later in the day I could have another cup of soup if I wanted. My vegetables should be chosen from the list of "regular use vegetables" and should include root vegetables, round vegetables, and leafy green vegetables. *Azuki* beans and lentils would be my main beans, and once a month I could have a serving of chickpeas. My beans should always be cooked with *kombu* sea vegetable. Bean products, like tofu, *tempeh*, and *natto* could be taken once a week, always cooked and in small amounts. I could have a small amount of homemade fermented pickles, and for thirst I could drink spring water, *bancha* twig tea, or barley tea. I was to avoid all animal products, including meat, poultry, eggs, and dairy food, all sweeteners, all baked flour products, and I was not to have any fish, fruit, oil, or nuts. A few special dishes were recommended, such as root vegetables cooked with a sea vegetable, and *azuki* beans cooked with *kombu* and squash. Shizuko told me how to prepare them.

I was to eat only when I was hungry and drink only for

thirst. I was to eat slowly and to chew my food very well. I was to go outdoors in the fresh air every day, and once or twice a day I was to massage my body with a damp cotton towel or a loofah sponge. As much as possible, I was to wear cotton clothing against my skin.

My kidneys were weak and overworked; my intestines, liver, pancreas, and gall bladder needed strengthening; my circulation was poor; I was anemic. Cancer was in my spine and my lungs.

"When should I come back?" I asked Shizuko.

She told me to call her in two or three weeks and let her know how I was doing. Then we would arrange another visit.

"What about chemotherapy?" I asked her. "Should I continue to take chemotherapy?"

My last chemotherapy treatment had been on February 16, when I was given two hundred milligrams of Cytoxan intravenously. My next appointment was scheduled for March 16, and I didn't want to keep it. I needed someone to tell me it was okay to stop the chemotherapy. No one would tell me that.

"You have to decide," Shizuko answered my question.

"What do you think?" I asked her. "Would it be better if I stopped?"

Shizuko looked straight at me. "Think, Elaine," she said. "Think what the chemotherapy does to your body. Think what the food will do to your body. Think," she repeated, "and then you decide."

I had one more question before we left. "Is there any hope for me?" I asked. "Do you think I can get well?"

She studied my face for a few seconds, and then she said simply, "You can recover."

* * *

The decision to continue or to stop chemotherapy was a

difficult one. Supposedly, the chemotherapy was killing the cancer cells. But was it, I wondered. I had taken various types of chemotherapy in varying doses for three years, and still my cancer continued to spread. Not only had the chemotherapy failed to reverse my condition, it had failed to stabilize it, to halt the steady progression of the disease. "Think of what the chemotherapy does to your body," Shizuko had said. I thought about what chemotherapy did to me. It made me weak, tired, nauseous, and bald. It reduced my physical mobility and my mental clarity. It caused vomiting, fluid retention, and bone marrow depression. It depressed my blood levels to the point where I had nearly died from a paper cut.

From my readings, I knew that Cytoxan can cause chronic lung problems. And Adriamycin can cause heart and kidney problems. My lungs were riddled with cancer. My kidneys were weak and overworked. What is the condition of my heart, I wondered. My cardiograms were normal—but so were my Pap tests when there was a tumor in my uterus, and my bone scan had shown a compression fracture when in fact I had cancer.

Chemotherapy suppresses the immune system, I knew. How could I get well if I kept weakening my immune system? How could I get well if I kept filling up my body with poisons? It didn't make sense. Was the treatment worse than the illness, I wondered.

"Think of what the diet will do to your body," Shizuko had said. The diet would halt the influx of artificial foods and chemicals into my system. It would cleanse my blood and strengthen my organs, neither of which would have to deal with a new arrival of toxicity every day. My body would begin to discharge the excess fat, fluids, mucus, sludge, and toxins that it had accumulated through the years. It would restore itself to a state of balance, and hence a state of health.

I knew that I would accept the macrobiotic diet. But I was afraid to stop the chemotherapy. Maybe I should do both,

I said to myself. I can stay on the diet and still take the chemotherapy every month. But I wasn't comfortable with that idea. That's silly, I told myself. The diet will take the toxins out, and the chemotherapy will put them right back in again.

"What should I do?" I asked Ralph.

"It's up to you," he answered me. "Whatever you decide, I'll support you. But I'm not going to make that decision."

"What should I do?" I asked Shayndee and Phyllis.

"Stay on the diet," they both agreed.

"What about the chemotherapy?" I asked them. "Do you think I should keep taking it?"

"You have cancer," they reminded me. "How can anyone tell you to stop taking chemotherapy?"

I didn't ask my parents. They had a lot of faith in doctors and in modern medicine, and I knew they would advise me to keep on doing whatever my doctor recommended. I didn't want to hear that. I didn't want them to tell me one thing when I was considering doing exactly the opposite.

I discussed it with Debra and Rachel. "What would you do?" I asked them. They didn't know. It was a big decision, a scary decision, one I would have to make alone. We could discuss the pros and cons, the fears and uncertainties, the benefits and the risks. But the ultimate decision would be mine alone.

"Think," Shizuko had said. I thought about chemotherapy. I thought about macrobiotics. And I thought about something else Shizuko had said. "You can recover."

I decided to stop chemotherapy.

* * *

My oncologist listened as I told her about the macrobiotic diet and assured her that it was nutritionally sound. Any diet is acceptable, she told me, as long as it provides all the essential components of good nutrition.

She did not think it was wise to stop chemotherapy, and she assured me that I would have no debilitating side effects from the small doses I would be getting. I explained that I didn't think that the small doses would do me any good, that if heavy doses of Adriamycin and CCNU didn't help me, what could I expect from two hundred milligrams of Cytoxan? I reminded her that I had taken Cytoxan before, and it hadn't worked for me then. Why should it work for me now when my cancer was so much more advanced? I had no confidence in it at all, I told her.

"I have a lot of confidence in this diet," I said. I explained that I was a firm believer in "you are what you eat," that other cancer patients had had success with this diet, and that I really wanted to give it a chance without chemotherapy.

"Let's go with the self-fulfilling prophecy," I suggested. "If I think the chemotherapy is worthless, it probably is for me, and if I really believe the macrobiotic diet will help me, it probably will."

She was not convinced. She probably thought I had gone off the deep end.

"Besides," I continued, "we don't have to commit ourselves to stop the chemotherapy. We can just delay it." I told her that if the cancer should spread further, I could always come back and take chemotherapy.

I tried to make it clear that I was not turning myself over to quack medicine. "It's just food," I emphasized. "There's nothing invasive at all, not even a simple blood test." I assured her that I had no intention of severing my ties with the medical profession, that I wanted her to continue to oversee me, that I had given the matter a lot of thought, and that this was really what I thought would work for me.

She saw my determination. She saw my disillusionment with chemotherapy and my confidence in the diet.

"I have no problem with delaying chemotherapy," she said much to my relief. And she went on to say that I should continue taking the Megace and that I should not forget to come back to see her.

The Megace! I had already stopped taking it. I had stopped taking everything. I had gradually reduced to zero the thirty-eight pills I had been taking every day. One of the benefits of macrobiotics was that I would not have to take pills. I hated popping pills, and I especially hated the Megace.

"I don't want to take any more Megace," I told my oncologist.

She felt very strongly that I should continue to take it. It was the only protection I had, it would not cause any side effects nor would it interfere with my diet. It was important that I take it every day.

"I already stopped," I confessed. "And I stopped all my vitamin supplements. And I feel better than I've ever felt in the past three years."

She was not angry. She did not dismiss me as her patient as I had feared she might do. She did not try to convince me that I was making a mistake. She was compassionate and understanding. She was human.

My oncologist would continue to see me regularly. My macrobiotic advisor would give me *shiatsu* and adjust my diet. I felt lucky. I felt grateful. I felt optimistic. I had two great women behind me.

* * *

Chapter 6

I AWOKE AND TURNED MY HEAD to look at the digital clock on the night table next to my bed. Seven A.M. I blinked and looked again. Sure enough, it was seven A.M.

"Ralph," I said excitedly when he came out of the shower. "It's seven o'clock!"

"I know," he snswered. "Why don't you go back to sleep?"

"Ralph," I said again, "It's seven o'clock in the morning and I was up only twice!"

"What are you talking about?" he asked me.

"I was up only twice," I repeated. "I woke up only two times to use the bathroom!"

"Only twice the whole night?" he questioned.

It was the middle of April, and during the past two months I had been getting up about seven or eight times a night, an improvement over my previous twelve times a night. I could now get off my hospital bed and, with the help of a walker or a cane and the walls, I could hobble over to the bathroom without waking Ralph. Before I looked at the clock this morning, I had thought it was the middle of the night and I was getting up for the third or fourth time.

"You probably didn't drink enough," Ralph said.

"I drink enough," I told him. "I drink when I'm thirsty."

He reminded me that I hardly ever get thirsty, and he told me, as he had been doing for the past two months, that I was not taking enough liquid.

"Remember what Shizuko said," I told him. "Not hungry, don't eat; not thirsty, don't drink."

"Shizuko doesn't have all the answers," Ralph said. "Everyone knows that it's important to drink a lot."

I told Ralph that when people eat meat and hard salty cheeses and other foods that impact in and around their kidneys and other organs, they have to drink to flush out the toxins. I told him that the kidneys are not meant to handle all the toxic nitrogen that results from the breakdown of animal protein. "Most of us flood our kidneys," I said. "We don't give them a chance to rest."

Ralph shook his head in disbelief. It amazed him how literally I was taking all this, and how much faith I had in it all.

"Have a good day," he said before he left for work. "And don't forget to drink enough."

I had no intention of forcing myself to drink. There's plenty of liquid in the food, I reasoned. When I cook a cup of brown rice with a cup and a half of water, that breaks back down to liquid in my body. Vegetables have a high liquid content, and I eat soup every day. I was feeling good. My stomach wasn't bloated anymore, and I had just had the best night's sleep that I had had in the past three years.

For the next week I continued to wake up twice each night, and by the beginning of May, I was waking up only once. I realized that I was urinating less often during the daytime too, and the intensity of the urge was greatly reduced. "You'll have to learn to live with it," so many doctors had told me for three years. Shizuko had no X-ray machine, she had no complex technological devices. She had simply studied my face and had known without a doubt that "condition can improve."

* * *

The art of evaluating a person from his facial features, or from the form and lineaments of his body, is called physiognomy. Physiognomy employs no elaborate, expensive, or hazardous technology. Each area of a person's face corresponds to an inner organ and its functions, and by using his senses, his intuition, and his judgment, the person experienced in this art can foresee the development of disease even before specific symptoms arise. By visual observation alone, an individual's past, his present, and his probable future can be determined.

Physiognomy fascinated me, and I was able to learn a little more about it in April when Murray Snyder, Director of the East West Foundation in Baltimore, came to New Jersey to lecture. Murray was tall, dark, and handsome, with a boyish grin and an enthusiastic personality. Like all senior macrobiotic teachers, he had been a student of Michio Kushi's for at least ten years. He was a dynamic and inspiring speaker.

Murray drew a large face on the blackboard, and as he filled in the features, he explained their correlation to our internal organs. The forehead represents the intestines, I learned, and the upper part of the forehead shows the condition of the bladder. The tip of the nose represents the heart and its functions, the middle part of the nose represents the stomach, the middle to upper part shows the pancreas, and the area between the eyebrows shows the condition of the liver. The mouth represents the digestive tract; the upper lip shows the condition of the stomach, and the lower lip shows the intestines. The area around the mouth corresponds to the sexual organs, and the condition of the lungs can be seen in the cheeks. The ears represent the kidneys, as does the area beneath the eyes. The iris and whites of the eyes reflect the condition of the entire body.

I sat in my wheelchair, fascinated, as Murray explained the meaning of a double chin, horizontal lines on the forehead, vertical lines between the eyes, a crease or cleft or swelling of the nose, bags beneath the eyes, and bumps on the head. He talked about spots, swellings, and discolorations, and he explained how various illnesses can be detected long before a person becomes symptomatic. He explained how the foods that we eat show up in our faces and how they affect our internal organs.

I was very impressed with Murray Snyder, and I was glad that I had arranged to see him the next day while he was still teaching in New Jersey. I put more faith in traditional Oriental evaluation methods than in a modern x-ray machine.

The next morning, Ralph drove me over to Hilda Sorhagen's house, where Murray was teaching. I sat in my wheelchair across the desk from him and gave him a brief summary of my condition, diet, and lifestyle. I told him that I had been practicing macrobiotics since February and that I was following the principles that Shizuko Yamamoto had given me a month ago. Murray studied my face and features. He asked me a few questions, and then he made his recommendations.

Pressure-cooked brown rice, every day; millet, three or four times a week; pearl barley, two or three times a week; sweet rice *mochi*, two or three times a week in soup; no flour products. Vegetables should be evenly divided among root, round, and leafy green varieties, always cooked. Three or four times a week I was to prepare a stew with root vegetables, three times a week I was to have *azuki* beans cooked with *kombu* and squash, and every day I was to have boiled or steamed leafy green vegetables. My soup should be cooked with *wakame* sea vegetable, my beans with *kombu*, and two or three times a week I was to prepare a side dish of *arame* or *hijiki* sea vegetable. A small piece of *takuan* (radish) pickle or *umeboshi* plum could be taken occasionally after a meal to aid digestion. I was to have no fish, no fruit, no nuts or nut butters, no spices, nothing raw, and nothing cold.

Karen Davis was in the room with us marking down everything that Murray recommended. She gave me the list. Murray had a picture of a face on his pad, and he filled it in with what he saw in me. I leaned forward and tried to peek, but I didn't understand what he was drawing. He gave me his phone number in Baltimore and told me to feel free to call him if I had any questions.

"I'm tired a lot," I told him, "and sometimes I feel weak. And I'm always cold."

He said that I was still anemic, and that some of the foods he had recommended would help that condition. He told me not to worry.

"So," I said as I was about to leave, "the diet will heal my anemia and my cancer."

"Oh no," Murray corrected me. "*You* will heal your cancer. The diet will be your tool."

* * *

On a sheet of white paper, I drew seven boxes and labeled them Sunday, Monday, Tuesday, Wednesday, Thursday, Friday, and Saturday. Each box was divided in thirds, and labeled Breakfast, Lunch, and Dinner. In at least seven boxes I wrote "rice," four boxes said "millet," three said "pearl barley," three said "vegetable stew," three said "*azuki* squash," and two said "sea vegetable." Every breakfast box said "miso soup," and every dinner box said "leafy greens." I filled in the remaining spaces with various grains, beans, and vegetables.

I attempted to cook and eat according to my planned menu. It didn't work. Before the end of the first week I was frustrated and depressed. I didn't always want what the box said. Monday night's beans weren't appealing for Tuesday's lunch, and by Thursday they weren't fresh anymore. Sometimes I wanted barley when the chart said millet, and sometimes I forgot to put *mochi* in the soup on the right day. The *arame* and *hijiki* I found offensive, and I could neither cook them nor eat them at all. I was developing a distaste for the rice, and often I had no appetite.

"I can't live like this," I said to myself. "I can't eat according to a chart."

I thought it over and made a decision. I would eat brown rice every day, and I would eat millet and barley at least a few times a week, as I had been doing anyway. I would try to eat everything that Murray had recommended, but not necessarily the suggested times per week, and certainly not

152

at a predetermined meal if the food didn't appeal to me at that particular time. Over the course of the week I would try to include everything, and if I was short a time or two on a particular dish, I wouldn't worry about it. I would consider my desires, my moods, and my appetite. I would allow myself to think—to think and to decide what I wanted to eat within the confines of my allowable foods. Only one thing was absolute—I would not eat anything that wasn't on my recommendations.

I tore up the chart with the twenty-one boxes.

* * *

On Monday, April 18, I felt extremely weak and tired. I stayed in my hospital bed all day; I had no desire to cook or to eat or to practice my walking. Tuesday was the same, and Ralph was worried. He reminded me that I had been feeling tired all week, and he wanted to take me to the doctor. I refused to go.

"You shouldn't be this weak," Ralph said. "You're going back to where you started. Maybe the diet isn't enough. Maybe you need some normal food."

"I eat normal food," I told him. "I eat only normal food. I'm just tired. It'll pass."

"Why won't you go to the doctor?" he asked me.

"Because she'll want me to take X-rays," I told him.

"Maybe she won't," Ralph answered. "Maybe she'll just want to examine you."

"What can she tell by examining me?" I asked him. "She'll probably suspect that the cancer is spreading, and the only way she'll be able to tell is with X-rays or scans."

"Suppose the cancer is spreading," Ralph said. "We have to know."

"We're seeing Shizuko next week," I reminded him. "Maybe she'll know and she'll tell us."

Ralph was getting annoyed. "I want you to go to the doctor," he insisted.

"I won't go," I said. "I won't go until after I see Shizuko."

"What about a blood test?" Ralph suggested. "I'm sure you're very anemic."

"I'm sure too," I told him. "So why bother with a blood test?"

"You can't just lie here like this," Ralph persisted. "Let's go for a blood test and see what the doctor says."

"She'll say to eat steak or liver," I answered. "Or she'll tell me to take iron supplements."

"Maybe you should eat steak once in a while," Ralph suggested. "You're probably not getting enough protein."

We argued back and forth. Finally Ralph said, "Go for me. Go because I want you to go. You don't have to eat steak or do anything you don't want to. Just take a blood test so that we'll know if the anemia is the cause of the fatigue."

I considered his request. It wasn't unreasonable, I decided, and it seemed to mean a lot to him. "I'll go on one condition," I told him. "Whatever the results of the blood test, we won't do anything without talking to Shizuko."

On Wednesday afternoon we drove to the hospital blood lab, and blood was drawn for a complete blood count. On Thursday afternoon I got a call from my oncologist's nurse.

"Your blood levels are critical," she said. "The doctor wants to see you first thing in the morning."

"I can't come tomorrow," I told her.

"You must," she said. "The doctor told me to tell you that it's very important for you to come in right away."

"My husband can't bring me tomorrow," I explained. "I'm in a brace and in a hospital bed, and nobody else is able to transport me. I'll come on Monday."

The nurse hesitated. "She really wants you to come tomorrow," she said.

"I feel okay," I told her. "Just a little weak and tired. I'm sure I'll make it until Monday. How low is my blood?"

She told me that my red cells were very low, my hemoglobin was very low, and my platelets were very low. But they were most concerned about my white cells, which were dangerously low. She told me to be sure not to come in contact with anyone with a cold or an infection, to stay away from crowds, and to be very, very careful. It would be extremely dangerous if I were to catch anything, she explained, because I didn't have enough white cells to fight an infection. We made an appointment for Monday afternoon.

I hung up the phone and called Shizuko. "Should I make any changes in my diet?" I asked her.

"Don't change anything until I see you," she said.

I told her that I had an appointment with my doctor on Monday afternoon. She agreed to see me on Sunday morning.

* * *

Shizuko gave me a deep and thorough *shiatsu*, using both her hands and her feet. I moaned and groaned at certain points, but the overall pain was less than it had been the time before. Again she took my pulses. "Not quite anemic," she told me, "but close, close." (I learned the next day that my hemoglobin count was 10.9—almost anemic.) Again we breathed together, as she raised and lowered her hands over my body while chanting, "breathe in, breathe out, breathe in, breathe out." I trembled under her touch, and I could feel the heat and vibrations between her hands and my body. I felt as if energy was being transferred from her into me. Was this palm healing? Was this faith healing? I had never believed in this before, I had never understood it, and I had never cared to. Now I was in the midst of this strange experience and feeling relaxed and comfortable with it. I felt as if I was being recharged.

I told Shizuko what I was eating, that I didn't have much of an appetite, and that I had developed a distaste for the rice.

"She doesn't eat sea vegetables, either," Ralph interrupted. "All she eats is a little rice and some plain vegetables."

Shizuko asked me what foods I enjoyed. I told her that I

liked most of the vegetables, but that I didn't eat too much because I didn't like the rice, and I didn't want to throw my proportions off.

Shizuko told me not to worry about the proportions for now. I could eat more vegetables if I wanted to, it was important that I eat. "Make a variety," she told me. "Every day, eat many colorful vegetables." She assured me that soon I would like the rice again.

"What about the sea vegetables?" Ralph asked. "She doesn't like the sea vegetables."

Shizuko told us that very often when people have eaten a lot of dairy food in their past, they have difficulty getting used to the sea vegetables. She said that I should try to eat a little, but if I absolutely couldn't, I should at least cook with them. She told me how to prepare a soup stock from *kombu*, and she recommended that I use it sometimes instead of water for cooking soup and grains. Every few days I should try to eat some sea vegetables, she said, and it wouldn't be long before I would be able to tolerate them. Soon I would even like them, she told me.

"What about my blood?" I asked her. "Suppose my doctor wants me to take iron supplements or vitamin pills?"

Shizuko didn't think I would need any supplements.

"What about a blood transfusion?" I asked.

She thought that a blood transfusion would not be necessary.

"Suppose my doctor wants me to take B_{12} or Folic Acid injections," I asked. "Should I agree to any medical treatment at all?"

Shizuko said that she didn't think it would be necessary. She said I could call her after I spoke to the doctor.

Because of the condition of my kidneys and other organs, she didn't want me to have any animal food yet. For my anemia though, and for my weakened condition, she recommended that I have a bowl of *koi koku* every day for the next ten to fourteen days.

"What's *koi koku*?" I asked her, mispronouncing the word.

Shizuko told me how to prepare *koi koku*. I was to buy a fresh carp and have only the gall bladder and the bitter bone removed. I was to chop the entire fish into one-half inch slices, including the head, bones, fins, and scales, and I was to cook the carp with an equal amount of thinly shaved burdock (root vegetable) for four to six hours in a pot or for two hours in a pressure cooker. A small ball of used *bancha* twigs wrapped in cheesecloth was to be added to the pot to help soften the bones. The dish was to be seasoned with *miso*, and I was to eat only one small bowl a day until the quantity was used up. This would increase my strength and vitality.

My kidneys were still stagnated, Shizuko told me, and they needed to discharge toxins. To help this process, she recommended that I apply a ginger compress every day to my back, behind my kidneys. She explained this process to Ralph, who was frantically writing down everything she said.

"Did I get worse?" I asked Shizuko, popping my face in front of hers so that she could look straight at me. "Did I get any worse since the last time you saw me?"

"No, no, no," she assured me. She told me to remember that I was very, very sick and that it would take time for me to get well again.

"You must be patient, Elaine," she told me. "Be patient and don't worry. Condition is better. You will recover."

* * *

My spirits were as bright as the sun, I felt no weakness or fatigue; I felt energized.

Was it the *shiatsu*, I wondered, or was it what Shizuko had said? The last time she had told me "You *can* recover," today she had said confidently, "You *will* recover."

"She said I will recover," I told Ralph happily as I hobbled back to the car on his arm. "Did you hear?"

Ralph reminded me that she had also said that I was very sick, that I was anemic, that my kidneys were still stagnated,

and that my other organs weren't in such good shape either.
I still had cancer. "Try not to take every word she says so
seriously," Ralph said. "She's only a human being."

"You're a pessimist," I told him.

"I'm not a pessimist," he answered. "I'm a realist."

"As long as we're in New York," I said to Ralph as we
approached the car, "let's stop in one of the big macrobiotic
natural food stores."

He looked at me as if I had just lost my mind. "You're
going straight home and back to bed," he told me.

"But I feel fine," I said. "I don't want to go to bed, I
want to go shopping. As soon as I start to feel tired we can
go home. Besides," I added, "we need some burdock for the
koi koku."

Ralph shook his head in disbelief. "All right," he consented,
"I'll take you shopping."

It was my first time in a store without my wheelchair. I
held on to the wagon while Ralph picked the various items
from the shelves. "Are you all right?" he kept asking me.
"I'm fine," I said, and when I started to feel tired I told him.
We went home and I slept soundly all afternoon. I had no
doubt that the anemia would soon recede.

When my oncologist saw me on Monday, the first thing
she said was, "You lost weight."

"Just a few pounds," I told her, "but I feel good and I'm
not bloated anymore. I'm much better than I was last week
when I came in for the blood test."

I told her that I had seen my macrobiotic advisor and
that she thought that the anemic condition would improve.
"I'd like not to treat it at all," I said, "and give it some time
to improve by itself."

My oncologist told me that ordinarily when a person
comes in with a blood picture like mine, it's very serious and
cause for concern. But because of the heavy chemotherapy I
had taken, and because chemotherapy sometimes causes a
delayed blood count depression, it was very possible that my

blood fluctuations were a result of the previous chemotherapy. She said that since I felt better now, we could just watch it for a while, and if the symptoms reappeared I should call her right away. She smiled and said that she knew that I didn't want to do anything that might interfere with my diet.

"How much weight did you lose?" she asked me. "How much do you weigh now?"

I told her that I had started my diet at 112 pounds and that I now weighed 101. "I lost eleven pounds," I said, "but I feel much better being a little lighter."

She told me that I shouldn't lose any more weight, and that if my diet wasn't satisfying enough I should intersperse it with some regular food. "You can be on the diet for three weeks of the month," she suggested, "and eat regular food for the remaining week." I said I would consider that, but I think we both knew that I didn't mean it.

We made another appointment for June, and she reminded me to call her if I had any problems in the meantime.

Ralph and I spent the rest of the week trying to locate a carp. My local supermarket didn't have any, and neither did any of the fish markets in the area. Evelyn called every fish store in the Yellow Pages, but nobody had carp nor could they order any. Finally, Ralph found a store not too far from his office, and they promised to have a carp for us on Thursday. They would clean it up and slice it for us.

"Call them back," I told Ralph, "and tell them not to remove the head, bones, fins, or scales."

Evelyn came over with her used *bancha* twigs, Ralph brought home the carp, and on Friday we prepared *koi koku*. We divided it into ten jars, and every day I ate a small bowl of it. The first few days it tasted delicious, then it lost its appeal, and by the last few days I didn't like it at all. I ate it anyway and felt stronger every day. When the last of the *koi koku* had been consumed, I felt better than I had felt before the whole incident started. The anemic condition never recurred.

*   *   *

In the middle of May, I took off my brace for good. I had been taking it off occasionally, first for an hour here and there, then for the night, and then during the day when I was in bed. Gradually I stopped wearing it when I sat in the wheelchair and when I practiced walking. Now I took it off for the last time. I had worn the brace for eight and a half months.

My walking was getting better every day. I had stopped using the walker and I was getting around with the help of a cane. Sometimes I didn't need the cane; by holding on to the furniture, the walls, and the counter tops, I could manage to hobble around the house. Occasionally I let go and took a few tentative steps on my own.

With the weather turning warmer, I tried to go outdoors every day. We kept a chair on the front lawn, and with the cane I was able to walk from the house to the chair. Sometimes I walked up and down in front of the house, and sometimes I would lift up the cane, take a few steps on my own, and then rely on the cane again.

On May 22, after I had walked a short distance with the cane, using it, raising it, and then using it again, I felt I could make it alone. I dropped the cane onto the lawn, and walked up and down the block—all by myself!

I had been practicing macrobiotics for three months.

*   *   *

Evelyn and I sat on my front lawn trying to diagnose each other. I really wanted to study Oriental diagnosis, and Arthur Jackson had recommended a book, *How to See Your Health*, by Michio Kushi. Debra bought the book for me.

Evelyn was as fascinated as I was. We examined each other's hands and face, referring to the book for every line, spot, or discoloration we saw. We took off our shoes and checked our feet and toes. The conclusion we drew was that neither of us was in very good shape.

"Let me see your ears," Evelyn said.

I pushed my scarf behind my ears.

"Why don't you take the scarf off and get some air and sunshine on your head," Evelyn suggested.

"I don't have too much hair," I told her. "It's growing, but it's growing slowly. I'm embarrassed for anyone to see me."

Evelyn said that I shouldn't worry about what people would think. I certainly didn't have to be embarrassed in front of her, she said, and nobody else was around now anyway.

"Take it off," she persisted. "It's a beautiful day. It'll be good for you."

I took off my scarf. "You've got enough," Evelyn said as she shuffled my sparse hair this way and that. "What you need is a haircut."

I thought she was joking. But she wasn't. She thought that if the scraggly ends were cut off and if my hair was shaped and brushed properly, it would be passable. It was almost June, Evelyn reminded me. Certainly a short haircut would be better than scarves for the hot summer months.

Evelyn called her hairdresser, who agreed to see me that same afternoon. "Can you do anything with it?" I asked her, removing my scarf.

"Sure," she answered. "We can shape it into a short pixie."

The scraggly ends were cut off and the remainder was tapered to my neck. It was boyish, but I had to agree that it looked cute.

"Ralph will love it," Evelyn said, as we admired the new me in the mirror. "You look so much better."

I felt so much better—and younger—and lighter. Though my scarves weighed only a few ounces, a feeling of heaviness was a part of constantly wearing them. Now I felt as if a load had been taken off my head. When I looked in the mirror, I

no longer saw "cancer." What I saw was a young woman
with a slim figure, a cute pixie haircut, and a smile that had
disappeared and finally returned.

I was liberated from my brace and my scarves. I felt happy.
I felt free.

* * *

As soon as Shizuko saw me on May 31, she said that my
face looked better. My *shiatsu* treatment was less painful than
the last time, but whenever she touched a kidney point, I
knew it. My kidneys were almost ready to discharge, Shizuko
told me, and she recommended that I apply a ginger compress twice a day for the next two or three weeks.

My diet was broadened. I could have bread now if I liked,
one or two slices a week of unyeasted sourdough bread. Once
a week I could have either *udon* (sifted whole wheat) or
soba (buckwheat) noodles. Occasionally I could have a small
serving of split peas, kidney beans, or other beans on the
"occasional use" list, in addition to my regular use of *azuki*
beans, lentils, and chickpeas. I was not to have lima beans yet,
and I was to continue to abstain from eating fish and fruit.

"What about *tahini*?" I asked. "Can I use that sometimes?"

Shizuko said that sesame butter would be better than *tahini*,
and she told me to use it very, very sparingly and only once
in a while. She recommended that I pour off the oil that rises
to the top of the jar rather than mix it in, and she said I
should continue to completely avoid all nuts and nut butters.

"She's losing a lot of weight," Ralph said. "Do you think
she's eating enough?"

Shizuko told us not to worry about my weight. She
squeezed my arms, my shoulders, and a few other parts of
my body. "A lot still has to come out," she said. "First we
make you skinny, then later on, you can gain weight if you
want."

"What about the cancer?" I asked. "Do I still have cancer?"

"Elaine, you have to be patient," she told me again. She made an analogy to a person who is trying to climb a very high mountain. When he stands at the bottom and looks up, it seems almost impossible. The top is so far away. But when he starts climbing, slowly but steadily he progresses towards his goal, until one day the top doesn't seem so far away any more. He needs only to keep climbing and be patient.

She checked my chest area again. "Is it still there?" I couldn't help asking. "Do I still have cancer in my lungs?"

"Condition still there," Shizuko answered me. "But not dangerous."

"Does that mean that it won't spread?" I asked her.

"Don't worry, Elaine," she told me confidently. "Cancer won't spread. The danger is over."

* * *

I sat in the driver's seat of our family car. A nervous Ralph sat buckled up on the passenger side. It was more than a year since I had driven a car.

"Are you sure you're up to this?" Ralph asked.

"Positive," I answered him. "I can't be dependent on you and the girls forever. I have to start driving again."

Slowly I drove down the block. Before we reached the corner, Ralph reminded me not to be nervous, to keep my eyes on the road, to use the rear view mirror, to put my blinker on, to look both ways before turning, and to be sure to tell him as soon as I felt tired.

We drove around town for about twenty minutes, and gradually Ralph relaxed. We did it again a few days later, and he wasn't nervous at all. I felt comfortable behind the wheel. I felt as if I had never stopped driving.

The next week I decided to venture out alone. I drove to a shopping mall about one mile from my house, parked the car, and walked into a store. I tried on and bought a cotton blouse, and I drove home again. I had reached another goal.

Evelyn continued to drive me to the natural food store. We had found a nice place to shop, Earth Things, in Rockaway, New Jersey, which carried a complete line of macrobiotic staples. The owners were pleasant, knowledgeable, and helpful, and they were genuinely happy to see my steady progression toward better health. The first time that we had come in, I was in my brace, my sweat pants, and my wig, and I had clung to Evelyn with one hand and to my cane with the other. Every two or three weeks we shopped, and each time I looked and felt better than the time before. By summer I was buying brown rice in twenty-five or fifty pound bags, and Evelyn was also buying brown rice, sea vegetables, *miso*, *umeboshi* plums, and other macrobiotic staples to use in her newly acquired pressure cooker. After our shopping trips, Evelyn and I often had lunch together.

Another friend, Evelyn Frank, who worked about two miles from my house, often came over and spent her lunch hour with me. Evelyn always ate before she came; she didn't want me to bother preparing lunch for her. Between her office and my house was a fish market and our butcher shop, and Evelyn often stopped there on her way over, assuring my family of a fresh meal of fish or chicken. For me she would bring either flowers, a plant, a stack of magazines, or a knick knack of some sort. When I was strong enough, we would sometimes spend the hour at the nearby shopping mall.

My friend Eunice, who lived on my block, was always popping over with something—a cotton sweater she thought was cute, an exotic salad for the family to try, a batch of cookies for Jeffrey to enjoy. Every day before she left for work, Eunice would call to see if I needed anything. On Saturday mornings, when our families were away at Synagogue, Eunice would come keep me company, and as spring turned to summer, we began walking up and down the block together. Our conversation usually revolved around food, and it wasn't long before Eunice, too, was eating brown rice, *miso* soup, and sea vegetables.

I was seeing my oncologist every two months, and in June I looked and felt much better than I had in April.

"What kind of miracles are happening here?" she smiled when she saw me. "Tell me what you're eating."

I told her I was eating a lot of whole grains, cooked vegetables, some beans, soups, and some condiments. I also told her what I wasn't eating—meat, poultry, fish, eggs, dairy food, fruit, sugar, or any refined or processed foods. I told her that I ate *miso* soup, brown rice, and sea vegetables every day.

"What's *miso*?" she asked me.

I replied that *miso* is a fermented soybean paste which contains protein, vitamins, and minerals, including vitamin B_{12}. *Miso* has living enzymes and microorganisms, I told her, and I explained that *miso* helps to neutralize toxins and discharge them from the body.

"Whatever you're doing, keep on doing," she told me. "Whatever you're eating, keep on eating."

On my chart she wrote, "DIET: MACROBIOTIC."

On June 28, I saw Shizuko again. My kidneys were better, she said, and I was making good progress. She said that corn was good for me now, I should eat a lot of squash, and I should have steamed greens every day. She recommended that I use lighter and shorter cooking methods for the summer.

"She's still losing weight," Ralph told her. "She lost twenty pounds already, she only weighs ninety-two."

Ralph was really worried about my steady weight loss. I knew that losing weight was a natural effect of the macrobiotic diet, and I regarded it as a positive sign. My body was discharging stored up excess—all the accumulated fat, mucus, and toxins were being released. The food I was now eating was being used for healing and for energy. I was using it, not storing it. So naturally I would lose weight until my body finished cleaning out.

"Not ready to gain weight yet," Shizuko answered Ralph. "More fat still has to come out."

"Where's the fat?" Ralph challenged her. "She's so skinny."

Shizuko explained that even though I looked skinny on the outside, I still had fat and accumulation in and around my internal organs. My intestines still had to discharge, she said. My kidneys were better but their cleansing was not yet complete. Also, other organs still had to discharge accumulated excess.

Ralph seemed doubtful. "Is it important that I eat three meals a day?" I asked Shizuko. I knew the answer, but I wanted Ralph to hear it from her.

"No, no, no," Shizuko answered emphatically. "Not hungry, don't eat; not thirsty, don't drink." She paused for a minute. "Listen to your body," she told me. "Body will tell you what it needs."

Shizuko thought that I needed to be more active. She suggested that I go outdoors and walk every day, barefoot on the beach, if possible, or barefoot on the grass. She told me that I could help stimulate my body by walking in place on a rolling pin, and she showed me how to do it. She also recommended that I scrub my body every day with a damp cotton towel or with a loofah sponge, ideally until the skin becomes red. This procedure would stimulate better circulation, she explained.

As she was planning to be away for much of the summer, we made my next appointment for September 7, right after Labor Day. Shizuko told me that I might have some symptoms of discharge over the summer, and if I developed a cold, fatigue, or some aches and pains, I need not be concerned. I was doing fine, she assured me, and I had no need to worry.

We said our good-byes and wished each other a good

summer. With no brace to restrain me, and no need to use my arms to support myself on a cane or to clutch at Ralph's elbow, I was able to give Shizuko a quick spontaneous hug, along with my thanks and endless appreciation for all she had done for me.

* * *

June had been a good month for me, but the happiest event of all was the day that Rhonda came home from Israel. Except for the week in February when she had come home for Jeffrey's Bar-Mitzvah, I had not seen Rhonda for more than nine months. During that time, I had regressed to the point of near death, and then reversed my direction and began the slow steady journey towards regaining my health. Although Rhonda was not with us physically, she was never out of our thoughts, and we communicated regularly both by phone and by mail. Excerpts from selected letters to Rhonda can describe, to some extent, our experiences from the time of my metastasis until June 1983.

October 4, 1982—from Ralph
" . . . I felt so bad last night after we hung up yet could do nothing about it. We gave all of the alternate ways of notifying you about Mommy a lot of thought, but there was no good way, and we decided to try to reach you as soon as possible. . . .

"I know how you felt, as I felt the same when the doctor called me in the office last Thursday. Debra, Rachel, and Jeffrey, not to mention Mommy, went through similar anguish, and somehow within a day or two we all managed to pull ourselves together and to look to the future with hope, as we did two-and-a-half years ago. . . .

"In the meantime, you can be our messenger in Jerusalem and do whatever you can to get our prayers to the right place. Keep a stiff upper lip and think positive. . . ."

October 12, 1982—from Ralph
". . . Things around here pretty much revolve around
Mommy twenty-four hours a day. As of today she has had
four radiation treatments. After tomorrow (fifth treatment)
we have an appointment to schedule her first chemotherapy
treatment, which is given intravenously in the hospital.
She has to stay there until the nausea, etc., dissipates. . . .

"Mommy's pain is at times pretty bad, and between the
effect of radiation and pain she is pretty weak. She still
can't lie down in a bed and when she does sit or sleep it's
on the living room recliner chair. . . .

"We have tried a number of medicines including two
different narcotic painkillers. Sometimes they work and
sometimes they don't. The doctors tell us that the pain
should eventually diminish after she gets more radiation. . . . "

October 13, 1982—from Ralph
". . . I hope you understand why I am doing all of the
writing these days. Mommy is very weak and can't handle
a pen or pencil. She, however, thinks of you all the time
and I'm sure deep down is somewhat sorry you aren't
around during this tough period. I remember around ten
days ago, when she was having severe back pains which
even strong narcotics wouldn't relieve, I was holding her
in my arms because she couldn't lie or sit and she was crying and asking me to bring Rhonda home. . . . "

October 17, 1982—from Ralph
". . . Last week was kind of rough, Rhonda. Mommy
finished her first round of radiation treatments on Thursday, and Friday she checked into the hospital for her first
chemotherapy.

"She has been terribly weak. . . . She can hardly walk
even when supported, as her legs are very weak. . . . The
nurse taught me how to give Mommy injections of vitamin

B_{12} and Folic Acid so she won't have to go to the hospital every day. I gave my first shots today and her backside is not even sore. . . .

"Mommy feels terrible that she is not able to write to you. First of all, she couldn't control a pen in her current condition and secondly, I think it's too emotional an undertaking for her at this time. . . .

"Anyway you look at it, it's a rough situation, Rhonda. You should, however, be assured that if I think you should come home I will say so. . . ."

October 17, 1982—from Debra
". . . Things here are so-so. Mommy is very weak. Let me apologize for her for not writing. She doesn't have the strength. It's all she can do to eat and go to the bathroom. I'm staying home tomorrow and Tuesday to help take care of her. I feel like it's a snow day—no work. I wish it were for a better reason. Keep writing Rhon—your letters mean a lot. . . .

"It's difficult to try to catch you up on what's happening with Mommy. It all happened so fast, and yet it seems like she's been sick forever. I'll start at the end by saying that now she's very weak, and has periods of bad pain. . . . She can hardly stand or walk by herself—she needs someone to support her. She's had five radiations and one chemotherapy so far. It's stronger than last time, which is probably why she is so very weak. It's scary and frightening—no one knows what the future will bring—but we all hope for the best. It can't hurt to be optimistic. . . ."

November 3, 1982—from Ralph
". . . Mommy's hair really started to fall out this week. She has a big bald spot on the back of her head. This time it will probably fall out completely. Debra had Mommy's wig cut at your beauty parlor (Princess Diana style) and I guess she'll start wearing it and her scarves pretty soon. She's still beautiful, and we are once again look alikes. . . ."

Early November—from Rhonda to Debra
Dear Deb,

Well, what can I write? To say that I'm doing great
and having a ball would be an outright lie. How can I feel
that way with Mommy lying in bed so sick? I'm depressed
and frustrated that I can't do anything. I'm scared and
afraid that I can't see what's happening to Mommy. I cry
a lot as I'm doing right now and sometimes I just want to
take the next flight home.

I'm also confused. You said, and Daddy wrote, that I
should "sound more concerned" in my letters. How? Does
Mommy really need to hear how I cry every night. Give
me some idea of what you are trying to say. I don't know
what to write. All I know is that I feel so far away from
everything and that I count the days until I will finally
return home in February.

I was so happy to hear that you're home a lot. Is
Rachel? How's Jeffrey? I also miss him so much, more than
I thought I would. How's he taking everything? Talk to
him, Deb. It wasn't so long ago that I was his age so I
know that he isn't a little kid anymore, so please make sure
he's not treated that way. I'm really concerned about him.
His Bar-Mitzvah is probably pushed to the side (which is
understandable) but still. . . .

Anyway, this letter wasn't to write about school, just to
tell you how I'm feeling—in short. Please send Mommy all
my love and please write soon and don't forget about me.

Send Daddy my love too (you may show this to him)
and tell him how much I *really* appreciate his detailed
letters. Make sure Daddy gets at least some rest from his
incredibly hectic schedule. I'll write soon again.

Your longing to be home sister,
Rhonda

November 15, 1982—from Ralph
". . . Rhonda, I read Debra's card—the card you sent
her recently. It made me cry. Rhonda, you need not be so

upset. I know it's hard being so far away and not being able
to be part of life at home. I'm writing you details as I don't
want to hide anything from you. As I wrote you earlier,
if (God forbid), I felt you should come home, I would
let you know. Hopefully you have experienced the worst
and from now on, with Mommy feeling somewhat better,
(from the radiation), you will also be less depressed.
Mommy and I want you to enjoy the time you spend in
Israel, and the last thing I want to be doing is upsetting
you. We at home have adjusted to the situation rather
well and you should do the same. . . ."

December 1982—from Jeffrey
    ". . . Things around here are not much different than
usual but I assume you don't really remember what usual
is. It's also a little different now with Mommy, but I've
learned to accept and get used to it and I'm sure you will
too. Last night Daddy and I went to a basketball game—
Nets vs. Knicks. . . ."

    February 22 to March 3, 1983—Rhonda home for Jeffrey's
Bar-Mitzvah.

March 1983—from Rachel
    "It's sort of hard to believe that you were ever home—
time passes so quickly. . . .
    "I suppose the most exciting thing happening is Mom-
my's new diet. She was already a little macrobiotic when
you were home, but now she's really into it. She had a
meeting with her doctor last week and told her all about it.
Much to all of our surprise, she wasn't against the idea and
said it was a good diet. Mommy seems to have a lot of
faith in this macrobiotic style, so let's hope it does what
it's supposed to.
    "Mommy and Daddy went to one of the head people in
this macrobiotic community—had an interview in the

city. The person (I'm not sure what one calls her) told
Mommy that if she stays on the diet things look good,
and her chances for recovery are good. I think her exact
words were, "You can recover." So as weird and foreign
as it all might seem to us—what the heck—it's sure worth
a try. . . ."

March 20, 1983—from Ralph
". . . Mommy is really thriving on her new diet. We
had an appointment with her doctor Thursday and she was
very understanding and agreed to keep Mommy off of all
chemotherapy, including Megace, until after the next series
of scans and X-rays. We were pleasantly surprised at her
reaction. She apparently believes that it is a nutritious diet,
and as long as Mommy is thinking so positively about it,
that it's worth giving a try. . . .

"Mommy really has been feeling good and is doing more
all the time. Let's hope this continues. . . ."

April 4, 1983—from me
". . . I'm still on my diet, Rhon, and it's working out
okay. Daddy and I are still going to cooking school. We
have two more lessons to finish the course. When you
come home, I'll cook you some macrobiotic meals. . . .

"Guess what, Rhonda? ? ? My hair is starting to
grow! . . . "

April 7, 1983—from Ralph
". . . Mommy's still macrobiotic and I'm still normal
and macrobiotic, that is I eat her food and everything else.
What a deal!. . ."

April 7, 1983—from me
". . . This Sunday, Daddy and I are going to a lecture
on macrobiotics. The head of the East West Foundation
in Baltimore will be in New Jersey on Sunday and Monday.

Sunday he'll be lecturing and Monday he'll be doing personal instruction. So of course I signed up for a personal visit, and I assume he will evaluate my condition and adjust my diet. I'll let you know. . . .

"I'm not wearing my brace in the house anymore, but I still put it on when I go out. This past Tuesday night I didn't wear it to cooking class, and Wednesday my back bothered me a little. So I guess I have to go slowly. . . ."

April 14, 1983—from me

". . . Sunday night we went to the macrobiotic lecture. It was excellent. Daddy and I both enjoyed it a lot. . . .

"Monday morning I had my personal interview. Guess what! I'm supposed to eat more sea vegetables. Ugh! . . .

"On Tuesday morning I went to the natural food store with Evelyn Ash and, among other things, I bought a fifty pound bag of brown rice! Would you believe? Rice keeps well, and now I don't have to worry about running out of it and trying to find someone to take me to the store. Also, they gave me a twenty percent discount. So I think it was a good idea—except now we have jars of brown rice all over the house. . . ."

April 16, 1983—from Ralph

". . . Mommy, except for being a little tired these days, feels all right. I guess if we ate brown rice and vegetables seven days a week we'd be on the weak side. She has lost a bit of weight and her stomach has really flattened out. . . ."

April 26, 1983—from Ralph

". . . The instructor in New York, Shizuko Yamamoto, or something like that, told Mommy she was sure she could ultimately get better and that the next few months may present some difficult times. She gave her a *shiatsu* massage, and indicated that Mommy's kidneys are still clogged and that I should give her ginger compresses. I

started this ordeal Sunday night. She also told Mommy to
eat more for strength, and she prescribed a concoction
which Mommy should eat every day based on carp fish,
including the bones, and vegetables. . . .

". . . On Monday night, we saw the oncologist who
feels that Mommy's low white blood count is due to the
effects of chemotherapy, but that unless Mommy eats better
she could end up being anemic which could cause problems.
She told Mommy if she doesn't like the macrobiotic food
she should switch off with normal food. She didn't say anything about supplements or tests, so we didn't either. . . .

"All in all, I guess Mommy's weakness is mainly due to
her not eating much and weight loss. She hasn't been
drinking enough either. . . .

"That's about all for the medical report—unless my sore
throat is of any interest. . . ."

May 8, 1983—from Ralph
". . . Today was Mother's Day and we had a little get-
together. . . .

"Mommy didn't touch any of the prepared food. She
waited until everybody left, and then she had rice and
vegetables. Everybody said Mommy looks well. Ever
since she has been eating the fish soup she actually feels
and looks better. . . ."

May 23, 1983—from Ralph
". . . Mommy continues to feel pretty good and this
week weighed in at ninety-eight pounds. . . ."

May 28, 1983—from me
". . . Yesterday I went to the natural food store with
Evelyn Ash, and today she took me . . . to get a haircut!
It's very, very short but the scraggly ends are off and it's
somewhat shaped. It's passable enough so I don't have to
wear a scarf all the time. . . .

"The Magnolia tree in front of the house is in full bloom. Spring is coming and soon you'll be home. . . . "

On June 13, 1983 Rhonda came home from Israel. We were a whole family again.

* * *

Chapter 7

I N PARTIAL FULFILLMENT OF THE REQUIREMENTS for the
degree, "Master of Science in Nutrition," it was necessary to submit a 7,500 word thesis dealing with a specific
approved subject. I spent the summer of 1983 researching,
studying, and writing my thesis, "Macrobiotics—An Alternative Treatment for Cancer."

A lot of thought and discussion had preceded my decision to
resume my studies towards a master's degree in nutrition.
Ralph had thought it was a good idea; it would give me
something to do for now, and it would result in a degree
which I could later put to good use if I chose to. Clearly, I
was interested in nutrition, and Ralph had thought I would
enjoy studying it again once I got back into the swing of it.

I had had a lot of reservations. It had been during the time
that I was studying nutrition, and practicing what I was
learning, that my cancer had spread to my lungs and my
bones. Is "health food," as we know it today, the right way
to go, I had wondered. Lean meat and poultry? Yogurt and
cottage cheese? Certified raw milk and fertile eggs? Raw
fruits and raw vegetable salads? Wheat germ and miller's
bran? Herbal teas and plenty of water? Vitamin and mineral
supplements? Protein, protein, and more protein? I had become disillusioned with conventional nutrition. I had discovered macrobiotics. It was working for me, and based on
what I was reading, macrobiotics was working for many
people— healthy people, people with minor disorders, and
people with cancer and other degenerative diseases. It was
macrobiotics that I had wanted to study.

Although I had been turned off by what is considered by

nutritionists to be a healthful diet, I could not discount the fact that my nutritional studies had given me a good education and a solid background that was now enabling me to better understand the macrobiotic way. I had studied anatomy and physiology—the structure and functions of the human body. I had studied organic, inorganic, and biological chemistry. I had studied the digestive system in depth, and I had learned about carbohydrates, fats, proteins, vitamins and minerals, their metabolic interrelationship and their role in normal human nutrition.

I knew that although the differences between natural nutrition and macrobiotics were many, similarities were also there, such as the avoidance of sugar and chemically processed foods, the reduction of fats, an increase in complex carbohydrates, and a return to a more natural way of eating. Perhaps, I thought, it would be possible to combine the two. Surely a knowledge of general nutrition could only enhance my understanding of macrobiotics.

My course work had been almost completed. It was the thesis that seemed like an overwhelming undertaking. And then—an idea had emerged! I would write my thesis on macrobiotics! I could complete my degree in nutrition and study macrobiotics! I could complete my degree in nutrition and study macrobiotics at the same time. It was an exciting prospect. Suddenly I couldn't wait to get started.

Donsbach University offered three modes of study—an on-campus program, an outreach program, and a homestudy program. On the homestudy program, I was able to complete my remaining two courses from my hospital bed. By summer, my thesis title and outline had been approved, I had purchased every macrobiotic book available, Ralph had bought me a comfortable outdoor chaise lounge, and I was ready to study macrobiotics.

We returned the hospital bed. I was able to sleep in a regular bed, sit in a regular chair, walk unaided, and drive a car. I continued to follow my dietary recommendations exactly; not a crumb, not a morsel of food that wasn't on my recommended list ever passed my lips. Despite the fact that my weight had dropped to eighty-eight pounds, I felt better and stronger with each passing day. All summer I sat outside on my chaise lounge, basked in the sun, and studied macrobiotics. At the end of August, I submitted my thesis.

I felt like a new person, renewed and rejuvenated. I was using my mind again, and I had accumulated a wealth of knowledge. I had changed drastically—from a sick, depressed, pill-popping invalid, to a happy, optimistic, pain-free, and very grateful woman. I had been practicing macrobiotics for six months.

* * *

When I saw Shizuko on September 7, she noted immediately that I looked better. It was clear that the cancer was receding, and it might be gone in about two months. Now I should eat a wide variety of food, I should include a lot of squash and pumpkin, I should eat greens every day, and I should also exercise more. She showed me some basic exercises.

"She can't do that," Ralph said to Shizuko. "She can't bend."

"She will bend, she will bend," Shizuko answered him.

"Try, Elaine," she said to me. "Every day, try to exercise. This is necessary for you."

I promised to try.

I gave Shizuko a copy of my thesis to read. I also gave her a copy of my case history to date, which I had recently written. I wanted her to review it before I sent it up to the main macrobiotic office in Brookline, Massachusetts for their records. We discussed my weight, which was now eighty-four pounds. Shizuko was not concerned and neither was I. But poor Ralph was convinced that I was going to just fade away and disappear. Shizuko assured him that this would not happen. I was doing fine.

On September 25, I saw Shizuko again. According to

traditional Oriental philosophy and medicine, the symptoms of cancer were gone. Now I was in a transition period. I should continue to eat more widely and to include more white vegetables. I should try to exercise more. I was too tight and I needed to loosen up.

I was seeing Shizuko regularly now during this transition period. She was doing much more than adjusting my diet to my changing condition and giving me *shiatsu* treatments. She was giving me encouragement, inspiration, and confidence.

At my visit of October 16, Shizuko again stressed variety. I needed a wider selection of grains and vegetables prepared in various cooking styles. I was exercising regularly, but not enough. I was still too stiff and inflexible. I must exercise more.

Shizuko suggested that I attach a before-and-after picture to my case history and send a copy to Michio Kushi and a copy to the *East West Journal*. She suggested that I also send a copy of my thesis.

Much to Ralph's relief, Shizuko said that I would soon start to gain some weight. I had lost thirty pounds. At eighty-two pounds, I weighed forty pounds less than Jeffrey, and exactly half as much as Ralph. I had shed thirty pounds of excess accumulation. Now I would rebuild my body with a variety of proper food. Real food: whole, local, and seasonal.

* * *

Every year, right after Thanksgiving, the *Whole Life Times* sponsors a three day exposition at a hotel in Manhattan. Lectures, panel discussions, and workshops are presented by leading spokespeople in the health field, including doctors, researchers, educators, and visionaries. One of the speakers on Friday, November 25, was to be Michio Kushi.

I wanted to attend the exposition, and I very much wanted to meet Michio Kushi. I packed up some grains, vegetables, beans, and snacks, and Ralph and I checked into the hotel for the weekend.

Michio Kushi looked exactly like his pictures—slender and wiry with jet black hair, glasses, and a warm playful smile. He spoke with a Japanese accent, and from my seat towards the rear of the Grand Ballroom, it was difficult for me to understand him. I had to concentrate on concentrating. After the lecture, many people came up to greet him, and I, too, pushed my way through the crowds in an attempt to personally meet the leading authority on macrobiotics.

Through the maze of people, I caught sight of Murray Snyder. "When did you get out of the wheelchair?" he asked as I approached him. Murray seemed genuinely happy with the progress I had made. We talked for a few minutes and he told me to be sure to tell Michio Kushi my story.

Michio Kushi and his wife Aveline were surrounded by people seeking information about macrobiotics, asking questions, and just wanting to shake hands. I was able to introduce myself and mention that I had recently sent them my case history. "Wonderful story," Michio said, and Aveline told me that my thesis was wonderful and I should continue to write and to study macrobiotics.

Although health food was available at the hotel, Ralph and I had brought our own and we ate dinner in our room. I warmed up my jars of rice and vegetables under the hot running water in the bathroom sink.

Ralph fell asleep before the next lecture on macrobiotics began, and as I didn't want to wake him or miss the lecture, I went alone. I looked around the room and saw Murray Snyder and Michio Kushi sitting together. There was an empty seat in their row, right next to Murray, and I took it.

Murray must have told Michio Kushi about me, because after a few minutes of conversation between them, Michio Kushi asked me if I would join him the next afternoon at St. Peter's Church. He would be speaking to a large group of people there, and he wanted to know if I would be willing to talk for a few minutes and share my story with the people. Of course I said "Yes."

Then I got a little nervous. I was not a public speaker. The last time I had made a speech was in college, when I gave a seven minute informative talk in a required speech class. I had written and rewritten that speech, I had rehearsed it many times, and I had still been nervous. What would I say to-morrow? I realized that I wasn't even sure of my condition now. I was changing so fast, and it was more than a month since I had seen Shizuko. I tapped Michio Kushi on the shoulder.

"Mr. Kushi," I said, "when I talk to the people tomor-row, what can I tell them about myself now? Is the cancer gone? Can I tell them I don't have cancer anymore?"

He studied my face for a few short seconds. "You can tell them," he answered me. "You can tell them that you are well."

* * *

I am well. In September, I had been told that the cancer may be gone in about two months. Now, two months later, this dream had become a reality. I knew that I was not completely healthy yet, that I still had a lot of internal housecleaning to do, that I still had to strengthen my body, that I still had a lot to discharge. But not cancer. There was no doubt in my mind that I no longer had cancer.

The speaker for the evening had not arrived, and Michio Kushi was asked to address the audience while we waited. I paid no attention to what he was saying; my mind was racing with thoughts of what I would say tomorrow. Suddenly I realized that Murray Snyder was nudging me. "You're on now," he was saying. "They're calling you up."

I snapped to attention. "What?" I asked him.

"Michio just called you up to speak," Murray said. "Go on. Everyone's waiting."

"Not now," I told him. "I'm speaking tomorrow."

I looked onto the stage. Michio Kushi was talking about a woman who had been very sick with cancer, and now she was going to tell her story.

"It's you," Murray said, grinning. "Go on."

"What should I say?" I begged him. I was feeling panicky.

Murray wasn't nervous at all. In fact, he seemed to be enjoying this. "Just tell them your story," he told me. "Tell them what you did."

I walked up the aisle and onto the stage. The audience applauded. Michio adjusted the microphone and stepped aside. I was grateful for the podium. I hoped no one could see that I was shaking.

"Hello," I said, "My name is Elaine Nussbaum. I'm not a public speaker. I didn't even know I'd be speaking tonight until just a few minutes ago." I spotted Murray in the audience. He was still grinning. Suddenly I relaxed.

My story came pouring out. Later on I realized that I had simply reiterated what I had written in my case history. Applause followed my presentation, and Michio Kushi came back on stage, shook my hand, and gave me a quick hug. I made it a long hug—I didn't want to let go. "Thank you, thank you, thank you," I mumbled, and I brushed away some happy tears as I stumbled back to my seat.

Murray pumped my hand and told me that I was a good speaker. Shizuko had arrived, we hugged briefly and then she held me at arm's length and looked at my face. "Good," she said unhesitantly. "You look good."

The next afternoon, as Ralph and I stood across the street from St. Peter's waiting for the light to change, I realized that I had never been inside a church before. More than three hundred people had registered to hear Michio Kushi's lecture that day. Many of them were cancer patients, some already practicing macrobiotics, some just beginning, and some still searching for a way to help themselves or their loved ones. I looked at the church. "Dear God," I said quietly, "we are all your children. Help me to inspire someone today. Perhaps

I can give hope to someone, perhaps I can play a part in saving a life."

Unlike the night before, I had no trouble understanding Michio Kushi's lecture. Afterwards, four people were called on to speak. A woman with cancer on one side of her head and face had refused disfiguring surgery and had saved herself with macrobiotics, despite her doctor's prediction that she would die without surgery. Another woman had freed herself of liver cancer. A man who had lost three-quarters of his stomach to cancer and had not responded to chemotherapy was now almost well. And me—a woman whose uterine cancer had spread to her bones and both lungs, and who was now well and flourishing in the macrobiotic way of life.

Again I hugged Michio Kushi. I hugged Murray and Shizuko. I felt an overwhelming sense of thankfulness. In the nine months it takes to carry a child, these people had carried me from cancer to health. Through their recommendations, their lectures, their writings, and their teachings, I had come to understand the macrobiotic approach to the cause and healing of illness. They had given me the tools with which to heal myself, and they had given me the hope, the inspiration, and the encouragement that strengthened my confidence and belief. Now I wanted to give back. I would share my story again and again, I decided. I would teach, I would lecture, and some day I would write a book. I would be grateful forever—to God and to nature, to my wonderful family, and to my advisors and teachers, all of who played such an essential part in helping me save my life and adopting a better way of living it.

* * *

I was a professional. My diploma hung on the wall, "Elaine Nussbaum—Master of Science," and I began seeing people in my new office that we had built from a part of our den. Many of my first clients were cancer patients, people who had heard about my own recovery and wanted to know about "my diet." My consultations lasted two hours, and in the cases of cancer or other serious illness, I recommended a follow-up visit with a more experienced teacher, usually Murray Snyder, Denny Waxman, Bill Spear, or Shizuko Yamamoto. As time went on. I developed a reputation. Friends recommended their friends and relatives, clients recommended other clients, natural food store owners recommended their customers, and physicians sometimes recommended their patients. I enjoyed my work immensely; I liked the feeling of being productive again, of being able to generate some income, and of helping people to realize a better way of eating and living.

As the story of my recovery spread in my community, people became interested in macrobiotics. "What do you eat?" I was asked over and over again. I quickly learned that most people thought it was impossible to put together a balanced meal without using meat, poultry, eggs, or dairy food. "What do you do for protein?" I was asked, and "Where do you get your calcium?" The fact that I had lost thirty pounds eating grains and beans never failed to fascinate people. Everyone wanted to know more about my diet.

I had become very friendly with Arthur Jackson, my first macrobiotic friend, and together we organized a series of macrobiotic cooking classes. Jacqueline Carboni, a certified macrobiotic cook, taught the classes. Jacqueline was wonderful, and everyone loved both her cooking instruction and her warm friendly personality. She taught family-style cooking, and it wasn't long before the word spread that you don't have to have cancer to benefit from, and enjoy, macrobiotic meals.

With a growing number of interested people, Arthur and I split up and ran two separate classes, one in Arthur's area and one in West Orange. People began to see results, the word spread that the food was good, and interest continued to flourish. In the year that I worked with Jacqueline and her assistant, Ken, we did twelve series of cooking classes, including elementary classes, intermediate classes, a class on cooking for children, and some macrobiotic discussion groups that included exercises and brunch.

Aside from developing a wonderful and lasting friendship with Jacqueline, I learned so very much from her. My notebook that was intended for the names and addresses of the cooking students quickly filled up with notes, hints, ideas, and information about the foods we were preparing. I was expanding my cooking at home, and I was gradually serving my family less and less "regular" food and more and more macrobiotic dishes.

By the end of December 1983, my internal organs were much improved. It was better not to have fish yet, Shizuko told me, but a little cooked fruit occasionally would be okay if I wanted it. Although I had lost another pound, I had regained it, plus three more. From a low of eighty-one, I now weighed eighty-five pounds. The *East West Journal* wanted to print my story in a forthcoming issue of the magazine, and Michio Kushi wanted to use my thesis for educational purposes and for publication. What a distance I had come since the beginning of the year, when in January, riddled with cancer, I had nearly died from a paper cut.

On February 19, 1984, Rachel was married. Just one year before, I had attended Jeffrey's Bar-Mitzvah in a wheelchair, a brace, a maternity dress, and a wig. Unable to walk or to stand alone, I had sat in a wheelchair and clapped to the music. Now, in a beautiful burgundy gown—size two—and in shoes that sported an attractive heel, I joined my family and friends and danced at my daughter's wedding.

I had been practicing macrobiotics for one year.

* * *

The rustic cabins were equipped with cots, electrical outlets, and showers with hot running water. Majestic shade trees, grassy slopes, winding hiking trails, and a sparkling natural lake were part of the campgrounds. Two full course macrobiotic meals plus a light breakfast were served daily, and a variety of educational programs and social activities were available. It was the eighth annual mid-Atlantic macrobiotic summer camp in the beautiful Pocono mountains of Pennsylvania.

Every June, macrobiotic teachers and friends gather together from across the country and around the world to share a week of educational and social activity. For me, it was an intensive learning experience. From early morning to late evening I attended exercise classes, cooking courses, workshops, and lectures. Others played softball, volleyball, and basketball, went hiking, swimming, and canoeing, or spent their time socializing and relaxing. I chose to study. I didn't want to miss a minute of any class; there was so much to learn, so much to experience. My macrobiotic understanding was greatly enriched, and I made many new friends, some just beginning macrobiotic practice and some long-time veterans. It was a wonderful experience, a wonderful week.

An idea that I had been toying with during the spring of 1984 came to fruition during summer camp. I decided to apply for certification as a macrobiotic teacher. I had been reading extensively and studying for almost a year and a half, and in my professional practice, I was providing macrobiotic information to my clients. I had accumulated a wealth of knowledge, and I wanted to formalize my studies, experiences, and counseling through certification by the East West Foundation and the Kushi Institute.

In order to qualify for the first level of certification, one has to have completed three levels of study at the Kushi Institute or the equivalent in independent study, must have been practicing macrobiotics for at least two years, and have been involved for at least one year in appropriate field work. Although I was a little short on the time requirement, I felt that I had the knowledge and the experience.

I had discussed my concerns with Jacqueline, who thought

that I should definitely apply. I had recovered from cancer, she reminded me, I had studied diligently, I had lectured, I had published, I was doing counseling, and I was assisting at cooking classes. "You're doing it," Jacqueline told me. Testing for certification was administered twice a year, in January and in August, and Jacqueline recommended that I take the exams in August. If I was not awarded certification, she told me, I would at least know where my weaknesses were, and I could study more and reapply in January.

I also sought the advice of Karen Davis. Karen was the certified macrobiotic cooking teacher whom I had met when she was assisting at the very first cooking classes that Ralph and I had taken together. Karen and I had become good friends, and I respected her knowledge and valued her opinions. Karen, too, thought I should apply for certification. She suggested that, in addition to my private counseling, it would be a good idea for me to spend some time assisting the senior teachers. I would learn a lot that way, Karen said, and it would certainly help to improve my evaluation skills, which was the area that I felt needed the most strengthening.

At the summer camp in June, I approached Murray Snyder. "I'm planning to apply for certification," I told him. "Could I assist you when you teach in New York this summer?" Murray said it was fine with him, but that I'd have to make the arrangements with Neil Stapelman, the managing director of the New York Macrobiotic Center.

Every week, from June until the end of August, I took the bus into New York and assisted Murray. Occasionally Denny Waxman came in, sometimes Bill Spear came, and I assisted them too, often spending as many as two or three days a week in the city. I saw many ears and noses and cheeks and mouths, I looked at many eyes, and I studied many hands. I listened to the teachers and I asked a lot of questions, and I learned an enormous amount. By the end of the summer I felt that I was ready for certification.

My son-in-law, Seth, was from Brookline, and his gracious

parents who lived just a few blocks from the Foundation, invited me to stay with them. My three days of testing included a written exam, a cooking test, an oral presentation, and an interview. While in Brookline, I was privileged to assist Michio Kushi in his personal way of life evaluations.

In October 1984, I received notification that I had been awarded first level certification as a teacher/counselor and a cooking teacher. Another goal had been attained.

My studies did not end with the receipt of my certification. When Jacqueline moved to Westchester to start a macrobiotic center there, I began studying cooking with Karen. Karen was an excellent cooking teacher with many years of experience. Her genuine concern, her gentle manner, and her healthful, youthful, glowing appearance were a real inspiration to everyone in her classes. I felt fortunate to assist her, to learn from her, and to further expand my understanding of macrobiotic cooking. Karen and I taught many series of classes in West Orange, and we planned for these classes to be ongoing. I continued to do private counseling, to assist the senior teachers, to lecture, and to write. Macrobiotics had become my way of life.

* * *

Although accurate macrobiotic dietary practice was the primary factor in reversing my illness, other considerations also contributed to improving the course of my recovery. Regular exercise became a part of my daily routine. In addition to the exercises that Shizuko had taught me, I was doing *Do-In* every morning. *Do-In* is a system of ancient Oriental exercises related to energizing physical, mental, and spiritual vitality. *Do-In* exercises are safe and easy, and they place little or no stress on the body. They can be practiced by anyone, in any place, in a short period of time, and I easily incorporated them into my daily routine.

After my diagnoses of cancer, I had stopped buying clothing

for myself. Why spend money on clothes, I had thought, if I won't live to wear them? Macrobiotics brought both a new attitude and a real need for new clothing. As my weight went down, I began to replace my mostly synthetic wardrobe with clothes made of natural fibers. Synthetics like polyester, acrylic, and nylon, which impede the regular flow of energy through the body, were replaced with cotton, linen, silk, and wool. My nightgowns, sheets, towels, and anything else that came in direct contact with my body were now made of pure cotton. Detergent and deodorant soaps and chemically perfumed cosmetics, which are damaging to the healthy bacteria on the skin, had been replaced with natural products.

In my quest for a more healthful and natural way of life, I turned to other macrobiotic way of life suggestions. I no longer ate in a hurry; I took the time to prepare my food properly and to chew very well. I discarded my aluminum and non-stick surface cookware and replaced them with good quality stainless steel. I used spring water for all cooking, and I drank only when I felt thirsty. I avoided electric, and especially microwave, cooking which contribute to undesirable effects on digestion and nourishment. I no longer took long hot baths or showers, which tend to deplete the supply of minerals in the body, and I added many green plants to my home, which freshen and enrich the oxygen content of the air and help to stimulate deeper breathing and stronger metabolism.

There was no doubt in my mind that my recovery was enhanced by my positive outlook and my faith in macrobiotics. A positive attitude enhances the immune system, which strengthens the ability to overcome illness. I believed that I could go from cancer to health through macrobiotics. And I did.

* * *

Chapter 8

For many years, evidence has been mounting linking cancer and nutrition. Prominent among numerous publications and pronouncements are two nutritional research studies performed for the United States government, *Dietary Goals for the United States*, in 1977, and *Diet, Nutrition and Cancer*, in 1982. These studies recommend sweeping dietary changes, including an increase in complex carbohydrates—such as grains, beans, fresh vegetables, and fruit—and a decrease in foods lacking fiber, such as meat, cheese, eggs, salt, sugar, fat, and highly refined and processed foods. Both studies concluded that our present eating habits are damaging our health, and that the suggested dietary changes can reduce the incidence of cancer, heart disease, hypertension, obesity, liver and gall bladder disease, and other bodily disorders. Given the wide impact on health that has been traced to diet, people need to be provided with dietary guidelines, and to be made aware of the effects of food on their physical and emotional well-being.

Macrobiotics derived its name from the Greek words, "macro" meaning "large" or "great," and "bios" meaning "life." It is the term used to describe a lifestyle that promotes health and longevity. Macrobiotics does not offer an identical diet for everyone. It offers a dietary principle that takes into account differing ages, levels of activity, levels of health, climatic and geographical considerations, and ever-changing personal needs. Macrobiotics is based on balance and harmony—eating and living in harmony with oneself, with one's environment, with nature, and with the entire universe.

The principles of macrobiotics are based on yin and yang, the two complementary opposite tendencies apparent in life and nature in endless variety and form. These principles are explained in detail in Michio Kushi's books on macrobiotics, from which the following synopsis is drawn. Yin and yang refer to the most basic, relative forces in the universe, expansion and contraction. These two forces are present in all phenomena, constantly attracting and repelling one another. Yin is the name given to the force that has an upward and outward direction and produces expansion. Expansion, dispersion, separation, dissipation, and wetness are yin tendencies. Yang is the name given to the force that has a downward and inward direction and produces contraction. Contraction, fusion, gathering, density, heaviness, and dryness are yang tendencies. Everything in the universe comes into being, develops, is maintained, and ultimately disappears as a result of these two primary forces.

Both yin and yang are present in everything, including our bodies and our food. An overall classification of food from the most yang to the most yin is: salt, eggs, meat, poultry, hard cheese, fish, grains, beans, land vegetables, sea vegetables, seeds, nuts, fruit, soft dairy, sugar, drugs and chemicals.

Some sicknesses are caused by an overly expanding tendency (yin), others result from an overly contracting tendency (yang), while others result from an excessive combination of both. In general, more yin illnesses are accelerated by the intake of more yin or expansive foods, such as sugar, dairy products, alcohol, drugs, and stimulants. More yang illnesses are accelerated by the repeated overconsumption of more yang or contractive foods, including meat, eggs, poultry, and hard salty cheeses. Some illnesses can result from an excess of both yin and yang extremes. When properly applied, the macrobiotic diet can help restore an excessively yin or yang condition to one of more natural balance.

The repeated overconsumption of food, especially food that

is extremely yin or yang, causes a variety of adjustment mechanisms in the body. Since the body at all times seeks balance, the normal process is for the excess to be eliminated, or stored when it exceeds the body's capacity for elimination. Normal elimination occurs through the process of urination, bowel movements, respiration, and perspiration. These processes take place continually throughout life. If we take in only a moderate amount of excess, these functions will proceed smoothly. But if the quantity of excess is large, the natural processes are not capable of discharging it, and various abnormal and chronic discharge processes begin, such as coughing, sneezing, heavy sweating, excessive urination, diarrhea, fever, allergies, and various skin disorders.

When the volume of excess exceeds the body's capacity for discharging it, it begins to accumulate, and internal deposits of mucus or fat begin to form in and around the organs. Since the lungs and the kidneys are usually affected first, their functions of filtering and cleaning the blood becomes less efficient, leading to deterioration of the blood quality.

The process of accumulation and degeneration can be reversed through a well-balanced diet that is free of toxic elements. By eliminating insulting constituents from the body, the process of accumulation can not only be stopped but actually reversed. The body naturally discharges excess food and liquid, excess protein and mucus, and excess fats and toxins that have been stored from years of accumulation of improper food.

Discharging is an important part of the macrobiotic experience. Sometimes the discharge process is so gradual that no visible symptoms appear. Sometimes temporary conditions do arise, such as general fatigue, aches and pains, light fever or chills, diarrhea or constipation, frequent urination, or skin eruptions. No special treatment is required; the discharge mechanism is part of the normal healing process and the symptoms should not be suppressed by taking drugs, resorting to vitamin supplements, or going off the diet altogether in the mistaken belief that it is deficient. In cases where these discharges become uncomfortable, a variety of natural steps can be taken to slow them down.

The macrobiotic diet contains an ample amount of all the necessary nutritional factors and provides them in their highest quality and most naturally balanced form. Many people believe that animal foods are the only source of protein. Protein is made up of amino acids. There are twenty-two amino acids in nature, and eight of them are called "essential" amino acids. It is necessary that we get these eight amino acids from food because the body does not synthesize them on its own. Any food containing all eight of the essential amino acids is considered to be a complete protein. Meat, eggs, cheese, and milk contain complete proteins, as does fish. There is also protein in grains, beans, and nuts and seeds, but these foods individually are deficient in one or two of the essential amino acids. However, the amino acids that are low or lacking in grain are abundant in beans, and the amino acids that are low or lacking in beans are abundant in grains. So by eating both grains and beans, one gets all eight of the essential amino acids—a complete protein. Grains and soy products, such as *miso* and *tamari*, also make a complete protein, as do the combination of beans and seeds.

Vegetable origin proteins are of a purer quality than protein derived from animal sources. Most animals are injected with hormones and antibiotics. They are forcibly fattened and artificially fed, and many of the chemicals added to their feed have been shown to be carcinogenic. These chemicals remain in the tissues of the animal to be assimilated later by the person who eats the meat. In addition, animal protein contains large quantities of saturated fats and oils, and it is now widely known that the unsaturated fats and oils contained in vegetable foods are more healthful than the saturated varieties found in animal products.

Protein is used by the body for growth and repair of the

cells. Our most efficient energy comes not from protein but from carbohydrates. Most Americans consume more than twice the amount of protein that they need. Excessive protein in the diet can result in accumulations of acids and fats in the blood, which tend to wash away essential minerals, such as calcium, iron, magnesium, phosphorus, and zinc. These minerals are usually leeched from the bones and the teeth to metabolize the excess protein, resulting in a weakening of the bones and the teeth. In addition, it has been reported by the National Research Council that a high protein intake is associated with a greater incidence of cancer of the breast, colon, kidneys, prostate, and pancreas.

Premised on the fallacy that the macrobiotic way of eating is based on a strictly limited variety of foods, some people have criticized it as being deficient in protein. In fact, between ten and fourteen percent of the calories on the Standard Macrobiotic Diet are derived from protein, exceeding the standard put forth by the Recommended Dietary Allowance (RDA) in the United States and by the International Food and Agricultural Organization and the World Health Organization (FAO/WHO). Even with a relatively limited caloric intake, the amount of protein eaten on a macrobiotic diet will approximate or exceed both the RDA and the FAO/WHO standards.

The people who live in Hunza, Pakistan and in Vilcabamba, Ecuador are noted for their health, vitality, energy, and longevity. They rely primarily on vegetable sources for their protein. Cancer is virtually unknown in both these regions.

* * *

The belief that dietary calcium must come from dairy food is largely a cultural phenomenon, unique to the United States and a few other industrialized countries. Throughout a large part of the world, dairy food is rarely consumed.

Milk is designed by nature exclusively for babies. No adult animal nurses from its mother or drinks the milk of another animal. Science and medicine have recently acknowledged that the human being, just like every other mammal in the world, is not able to digest milk perfectly after babyhood. This is because of a decrease in the enzyme lactase in the gastrointestinal tract. It is natural to lose this lactase activity; it is a biological accompaniment of growing up.

Good sources of calcium on the macrobiotic diet include sea vegetables, leafy green vegetables, beans, and nuts. Whereas one cup of milk contains three hundred milligrams of calcium, one cup of cooked leafy greens (mustard, collard, turnip) also contains between two and three hundred milligrams of calcium, and one cup of cooked sea vegetables (*kombu, wakame, hijiki*) contains between three and six hundred milligrams of calcium. Other vegetable sources of calcium include *daikon* watercress, dandelion greens, dulse, sesame seeds, soyfoods (tofu, *tempeh*), and *shiso* leaves. The calcium requirements for non-animal-food eaters is substantially lower than the requirements for those who do eat animal food, as the non-animal-food eaters do not accumulate the acid in their blood that leeches calcium from their teeth and bones.

In countries where calcium is obtained from vegetable sources, tooth decay and bone fractures are rare. Osteoporosis, the disease often regarded as being a result of calcium deficiency, is relatively common in industrialized countries and occurs less frequently in the Third World where dairy foods are not widely consumed.

Anemia is one of the most widespread nutritional deficiency diseases in the United States. This can be attributed to the highly refined nature of the American diet. Since the macrobiotic diet includes as one of its principles the consumption of whole and unrefined foods, it contains as much or more iron as its American counterpart. In addition to being present in whole grains, ample amounts of iron are found in beans, seeds, leafy green vegetables, and sea vegetables. Other

vegetable foods, including whole millet, *azuki* beans, chickpeas, lentils, pumpkin seeds, sesame seeds, barley (*mugi*) and
soybean (*hatcho*) miso, and buckwheat noodles (*soba*) contain
more iron per hundred grams than beef, eggs, and cow's
milk, which contains only a slight trace of this mineral. Sea
vegetables such as *wakame*, *arame*, *hijiki*, *kombu*, and dulse are
particularly rich sources of iron.

Although not a familiar food in our culture, sea vegetables
are included in the diets of many people throughout the
world. The large variety of edible sea vegetables provides
one of the best vegetable sources of minerals, plus a full com-
plement of protein and vitamins. All of the necessary vitamins, including vitamin C and B_{12}, are provided in proper
balance in the macrobiotic diet.

Some of the many foods rich in vitamin C include broccoli,
cauliflower, squash, cabbage, watercress, parsley, collards,
and kale. Only a relatively small portion of lightly cooked
vegetables, for example half a cup of kale, approaches or
exceeds the RDA and the FAO/WHO standards for vitamin
C. With regard to vitamin B_{12}, recent studies have shown
that this vitamin exists in suitable quantities in fermented
foods such as *miso*, *natto*, and especially *tempeh*. Contrary to
popular belief, it is not necessary to eat animal foods such
as meat or eggs to obtain the proper quantities of this or
any other vitamin.

As long as the principles of macrobiotics are applied in
choosing one's diet, nutritional deficiencies will not be a
problem. In a world where the incidence of degenerative
disease and general poor health is growing, the macrobiotic
diet is a sensible alternative to our overprocessed and de-
vitalized foods. It is a common sense approach to eating.

* * *

According to the American Cancer Society, thirty percent
of the American population, or close to one out of three

people, is expected to get cancer in his lifetime. Each year more than 850,000 new cancers are diagnosed, and approximately 450,000 people die of the disease.

Since 1971, the National Cancer Institute has spent more than seven billion dollars on its "war" on cancer. In 1979, for the first time in history, more than one billion dollars was spent. In that same year, 70,000 more Americans died of cancer than when the "war" began eight years earlier. According to the American Cancer Society, a cancer patient treated by conventional methods has a one-in-three chance of surviving for five years after diagnosis—exactly the same odds that faced a cancer patient in 1950.

Other degenerative illnesses are also widespread. Forty-two million people in this country have cardiovascular disorders, thirty-seven million have high blood pressure, eleven million are diabetic, thirteen million have birth defects, two million have epilepsy, and one-half million have multiple sclerosis. Fourteen to twenty-eight million Americans suffer from alcoholism, and tens of millions from abuse drugs. The rate of mental illness has increased substantially.

Until modern times, unrefined, naturally produced whole cereal grains comprised humanity's primary food world-wide, while locally grown seasonal vegetables comprised the most important secondary foods. People ate that which was grown in the same area that they lived. Today, though we live in the temperate climates of North America, we eat tropical and semi-tropical products (citrus fruit, bananas, sugar, coffee, spices), and we consume heavy animal food. We refine our grains and we adulterate our food with a myriad of colorings, flavorings, stabilizers, emulsifiers, deodorizers, sprays, polishes, and preservatives. And then we wonder why our health continues to deteriorate. Or we blame God for our illnesses.

The human body was not created to eat quantities of meat. Our teeth suggest their use for grain eating. We have twenty molars for grinding grain, eight incisors for cutting vegetable foods, and only four canine teeth for tearing animal food. Our long digestive systems are not meant to handle meat.

Grains and vegetables remain in the stomach for about two to two-and-a-half hours, whereas meat remains up to four-and-a-half hours. Animal proteins begin to decompose as soon as the animal has been killed. Although this process is somewhat retarded by refrigeration and the addition of preservatives, it resumes as soon as the meat is eaten, and is usually well underway by the time the food reaches the intestines. The putrefacation of animal protein in the intestines destroys the beneficial bacteria which synthesize the vitamin B complex that is utilized in the metabolism of carbohydrates and in the synthesis of glutamic acid in the brain. The putrefacation of animal protein causes body odor and odorous bowel movements. Excess animal protein results in excess body hair in both men and women. Excess animal protein turns into fat, which is stored first in the adipose tissues and then in and around the vital organs, causing them to enlarge and harden and to lose their ability to function properly.

Because meat is low in fiber, its travel time through the intestines is prolonged, and the remnants, fecal matter, remain in the colon for three and four days at a time. The putrefactive bacteria in the colon attacks the bile acids necessary for the breakdown of fat and convert them into powerful cancer-causing chemicals. These potentially lethal chemicals accumulate in the colon as each day passes. The fecal mass and its store of cancer chemicals may remain in the colon for days, continuously converting harmless bile acids into cancer-producing compounds.

The food of people on high-fiber diets (grains, vegetables, beans, seeds) takes approximately twenty-four hours to pass through the *entire* digestive tract. Fecal matter remains in the colon for less than eighteen hours. Bile acid in the feces is passed almost unchanged and intact, unaffected by putrefactive bacteria. The incidence of colon cancer in the United States is nine hundred percent greater than that of Nigeria and thirteen hundred percent greater than Uganda, two countries with traditional high-fiber diets.

Why do we drink cow's milk? Cow's milk was intended to nourish calves. It is the indispensable food for calves before they have teeth. When young animals have their teeth and are weaned from nursing, they no longer drink milk. Ever. Nor does any animal drink the milk of another species. Ever. It is biologically unnatural.

People are not cows. We do not grow like cows, we do not act like cows, we do not think like cows. There is no reason for human beings to drink the milk of another mammal —especially an animal inferior to him both biologically and intellectually.

Milk is often described as a near-perfect food, yet it is far from perfect. Cows on modern farms are often poorly fed. They receive toxic doses of antibiotic drugs both in their food and by injection, and many are afflicted with various diseases. So much residual penicillin has remained in some milk that the cheese industry has found the milk useless as a starter culture.

Much of the nutritional value in milk is destroyed through the process of pasteurization. The synthetic vitamin D that is added to milk gives toxic reactions in animal feeding tests. The homogenization of milk breaks down the fat particles and releases an enzyme called xanthine oxidase, which destroys vital body chemicals that would normally protect the arteries of the heart. It has been noted that the death rate from heart disease in different countries is proportional to how much homogenized milk people drink.

Dairy food affects every organ in the human body. Because it is a product of the mammary gland, it mostly affects the human glands and related structures, especially the reproductive organs. The most commonly affected are the breast, uterus, ovaries, prostate, thyroid, nasal cavities, pituitary gland, the cochlea in the ear, and the cerebral area surrounding the midbrain. Many of our current health problems are linked to dairy consumption, including vaginal discharges, ovarian cysts, fibroid tumors, breast tumors, many skin diseases, allergies, stone formations, hay fever, and arthritis.

All of these diseases are on the increase as dairy consumption continues to skyrocket.

But isn't milk natural? Cow's milk is a natural food for calves; the proportion of carbohydrates, fats, and proteins in cow's milk are in natural balance for a calf to grow quickly into a cow, not for a human baby to grow into a healthy adult.

Another contributor to degenerative health is the high consumption of refined sugar. Eating refined sugar is worse than eating nothing. Real food contains vitamins and minerals which help to digest and absorb it. Since refined sugar contains no nutrients, it drains and leeches vitamins and minerals from the body, resulting in a depletion of zinc, chromium, manganese, B vitamins, and other nutrients necessary for sugar's metabolism.

Refined sugar produces an over-acidic condition in the blood, and the body requires minerals to return the blood to a normal acid-alkaline balance. Sodium, potassium, and magnesium are drawn from the body, and calcium is taken from the bones and the teeth.

In the normal digestive process, complex sugars (from grains, vegetables, beans, and so on) are decomposed by saliva in the mouth, further broken down in the stomach, and finally digested in the intestines. The sugar is released into the bloodstream over a period of several hours. Simple sugars do not go through this digestive process; they go immediately and very rapidly into the bloodstream, making it difficult for the body to balance it with the proper insulin response. Excess insulin is released from the pancreas, causing excess sugar to be removed from the blood, resulting in "low blood sugar." If more refined sugar is taken at this time—which it usually is because the person feels hungry, weak, nervous, and irritable—the procedure is repeated, resulting in an overworked pancreas that may eventually become too weak to produce an adequate amount of insulin.

Excess sugar is carried by the bloodstream to the liver,

where it is stored in the form of glycogen. When the amount of glycogen exceeds the liver's storage capacity, it is released back into the bloodstream in the form of fatty acids, which are attracted to the heart and the kidneys. Fat and mucus eventually surround and penetrate these organs, weakening their normal functioning.

Refined sugar destroys the intestinal bacteria which are responsible for the creation of the B vitamins necessary for the synthesis of glutamic acid. Glutamic acid is the key to orderly brain functions. It is directly involved in the mental activities of the brain, affecting our ability to calculate, to remember, and to think clearly.

But isn't sugar pure? Refined sugar is pure to the extent that it is devoid of vitamins, minerals, and proteins; it is pure calories. Refined sugar is a highly processed product of tropical climates that ultimately affects every organ in the body, resulting in the degeneration of our physical, mental, and emotional health.

* * *

Chapter 9

O N AUGUST 10, 1984, I reached my forty-fifth birthday.
Forty relatives and friends who had helped and
supported me during my illness and recovery joined
us in joyful celebration with a macrobiotic buffet dinner.
It was truly a landmark occasion for me—to reach this birthday
that I had thought I would not live to see.

Ralph and I cooked all day. Our guests enjoyed hors
d'oeuvres of vegetables with chickpea dip, *tamari* roasted
pumpkin and sunflower seeds, assorted dried fruits, and
freshly popped popcorn. Dinner was an appetizing spread of
fried rice with *shiitake* mushrooms and onions, *azuki* beans
with *kombu* and squash, pasta salad, *seitan* stew, bulgur salad,
sautéed fish fillets with scallions and snow peas, assorted *nori*
rolls, a large tossed salad, and corn-on-the-cob. Blueberry
kanten, peach crisp, and *bancha* tea completed our party. Once
again, I can entertain.

On Thanksgiving 1984, one year after I saw Michio Kushi
and realized that I no longer had cancer, Ralph and I took a
week-long vacation in the Caribbean, where we enjoyed
delicious meals at a beautiful macrobiotic resort. In January
1985, we spent a long weekend in Chicago, where I managed
to cook some fresh food in addition to the prepared dishes
that I took along, and in August, we spent a few days at the
Jersey shore. With a little planning, advance preparation, and
some macrobiotic non-perishable staples such as *miso, tamari,*
sea vegetables and *umeboshi* plum, I can enjoy a vacation and
still eat reasonably well. Once again, I can travel.

Throughout the year, we have attended weddings, Bar-
Mitzvahs, dinner parties, barbecues, and various social gather-

ings. Depending on the circumstances, I either eat before-hand, bring along my own food, or eat selectively from the food being offered. Sometimes I do all three. To the best of my knowledge, I have never been left out because of my eating style. Once again, I can socialize.

When I spend a day in New York city, I often have lunch or dinner at a macrobiotic restaurant. When Ralph and I go out to eat alone, with the family, or with friends, we choose a restaurant with a selection of good quality natural food. When business associates need to be entertained, we take them to dinner and I order selectively. Once again, I can eat out in a restaurant.

Although I did not have the luxury of time, my family was able to ease into better eating habits on a gradual basis. In the beginning, we had "my food" and "their food." It did not take long to realize that macrobiotic soups are delicious, and we began eating the same soups. Why should I feed my family vegetables that are weakening while I eat the pre-ferred vegetables, I wondered. We began eating the same vegetables. Before long we were eating the same dinner every night, with the addition of a "protein dish" for the family. My main course would be grain, while they treated the grains like another side dish. It took a long time to eliminate the protein dish. "Rice and vegetables" did not adequately answer the question, "what's for dinner?" As my health improved and my cooking expanded, I began preparing "main dishes" for the family. The meals then had a name, and "what's for dinner?" could be answered with, "Peking fried rice," "barley casserole," "*seitan* stew," "millet loaf," "bul-gur croquettes," "noodle casserole," or whatever label I could attach that sounded appetizing. Red meat disappeared, and chicken was relegated to Friday nights and holidays. Cheese was easily eliminated, yogurt took longer, and milk was slowly replaced with *amazake* (a sweet beverage made from fermented sweet rice) and soy milk.

My family has made radical changes in their eating habits,

some members more than others. But even more important
than what my children eat, is what they have learned. They
have learned that there is an order to life, that things don't
"just happen." They have learned to understand the root-
cause of their physical and emotional well-being. They recognize the body's self-healing powers, and they do not turn to
chemical medication to suppress the symptoms of illness.
They no longer think of sickness as being a terrible thing
that happens to people at random, and they do not feel vulnerable to the ravages of degenerative disease. They have
learned to take responsibility for their own health.

My sisters Shayndee and Phyllis are also reaping the benefits of macrobiotics. From my recovery they discovered the
power of food, and they assessed their own dietary habits.
Though never diagnosed medically with a serious health
problem, they began to question the direction in which they
were going. Now they are eating macrobiotically, improving
their health, and ensuring themselves of a healthy future.
Their families are now being served foods that promote well-
being, and we are once again swapping recipes.

Through their relationships with me and their exposure to
macrobiotic cooking classes, many of my friends have made
changes in their own and in their families' eating patterns.
Some have changed from white rice to brown, from refined salt
to sea salt, from frozen vegetables to fresh, from commercial
tea to *bancha*. Some are eating whole grains regularly, some
are cooking with *miso*, sea vegetables, and *umeboshi* plum, and
many have drastically reduced their intake of meat, dairy,
sugar, and chemicalized food. Many of my clients who continue to see their physicians are having their progress confirmed by medical diagnostic procedures.

Some people claim that the macrobiotic diet doesn't work
for them. They take two or three cooking classes (family
style), eat brown rice (boiled) a few times a week, call themselves macrobiotic, and claim that the diet doesn't work. Some
people with cancer cheat "just sometimes"; on the weekends,

when they eat out, when they entertain, and when they don't have time to cook. Then they wonder why they do not improve. People who are in general good health and want to maintain or improve their health can usually eat a Standard Macrobiotic Diet and do well. People who want to heal themselves of a condition as serious as cancer really need to see a qualified macrobiotic instructor who will adjust the diet to their individual needs and impress upon them the importance of practicing accurately.

Many people ask me why there is no scientific analysis or statistical evidence regarding the success rate for the macrobiotic diet in cases of cancer. Record keeping is difficult for several reasons. Some people, after being told by the medical profession that they no longer have cancer, do not report back to their macrobiotic teacher. Others, who get better while practicing macrobiotics, do not return to their doctors for the medical tests necessary to confirm their recovery. Some people cheat on the diet, and when they don't make progress they claim that the diet doesn't work. Many patients start macrobiotics after having had surgery, chemotherapy, and/or radiation, and there is no proof as to whether the treatments, the diet, or a combination of both were effective in producing their recovery.

For many years, the East West Foundation has been working without the thought of making statistical information available. It has been more concerned with helping people than with keeping records. However, to meet the growing demand for this type of information, studies are now being conducted and records are being kept, and statistical information should become available in the near future.

Because something has not been scientifically proven, does not mean that it is not true. The approach is not harmful. It's just real food. One has nothing to lose but his illness.

*   *   *

When I decided to write this book, I gave thought to including medical documentation of my recovery. I decided against it. X-rays are weakening to the body, I knew, and I did not want to be injected with radioactive dye. Those who will believe will believe with or without X-rays, I thought, and the skeptics who will claim "spontaneous remission," or "previous chemotherapy," will also do so with or without X-rays. The fact is, there is no case of spontaneous remission of disseminated uterine sarcoma, and there is no cure with or without chemotherapy and radiation. The medical literature shows that there are no survivors.

When I asked my oncologist what percentage of patients recover from the type of cancer that I had, her immediate reply was, "as close to zero as you can get."

Still I pondered. I knew that many sick people might consider a macrobiotic approach as a result of reading this book. Might they need medical documentation to inspire them? Might their families need medical documentation to support them? Might their physicians need medical documentation to permit them? Might their friends and relatives need medical documentation to encourage them? Might medical documentation be necessary to convince them of my recovery?

On February 19, 1985, after two years of macrobiotic practice, during which time I took no drugs, medication, hormones, antibiotics, painkillers, tranquilizers, sedatives, cold suppressants, fever reducers, aspirin, or vitamin pills, I returned to the hospital for a complete set of X-rays of my spine and my lungs. I made an appointment with my oncologist a few days later to discuss the results of the tests.

"Here comes my miracle," my oncologist smiled at me when Ralph and I came into her office.

"I'm not surprised," I responded. "I knew what the results would be."

"I'm not surprised either," she admitted, and she showed me the initial report from the radiology department.

There was no cancer in my lungs or my bones.

My medical records state: "Frontal and lateral views at this time fail to reveal any definite pulmonary nodules. No infiltrates are seen in the lungs. No hilar or mediastinal adenopathy can be identified. No pleural fluid is seen. The cardiovascular silhouette is normal."

A subsequent comparison study of my 1985 with my 1983 chest X-rays revealed that there may be a tiny residual scar where a large tumor had previously been seen. "Regarding the chest, previously noted bilateral pulmonary nodules have *dramatically receded* since 1/18/83."

Whereas the old compressions of my lumbar and thoracic vertebrae are still evident, "No lesions are seen." The old tumors are gone, and "No additional lytic or blastic lesions are seen."

There was no cancer in my body.

* * *

After three years of macrobiotic practice, I remain healthy and productive. My nutritional practice has grown, and I have the satisfaction of helping many people to realize a better way of life through the proper quality, quantity, and combination of well-prepared food, regular exercise, and a positive mental outlook. I have written articles for several magazines, and I have lectured to various groups about macrobiotics. I continue to teach cooking classes with Karen, and I continue to learn from her. As time permits, I assist the senior teachers at the center in New York, and I continue to expand my macrobiotic knowledge and experience.

People have told me that I am lucky, lucky that macrobiotics worked for me. Maybe it was luck, or fate, that I discovered macrobiotics precisely when I had to find an alternative. Or maybe it was precisely because I needed an alternative, that I discovered macrobiotics. That it worked for me was more than luck. It was faith, determination, and accurate practice. It was gratitude and appreciation. It was

love and support from my family and close friends. It was
the realization that I was the cause of my illness, and I was
the only one who could reverse it. No diet alone can cure
cancer. No chemotherapy can cure cancer. The body heals
itself. As Murray Snyder told me when I was just beginning, "*You* will heal your cancer. The diet will be your tool."

I am no longer eating the strictly limited diet necessary to
recover from serious illness. Now I eat to maintain my health
and energetic activities; I include a wide variety of food from
all categories of the Standard Macrobiotic Diet. I love the
food, and to the relief of my family, I have gained ten pounds.
I enjoy good health, good energy, and good bodily functions. My memory, my judgment, my instincts, and my
intuition have all improved. There is no doubt in my mind
that I am a healthier person now than I was before my diagnosis of cancer. Through macrobiotics I have regained my
health—physically, mentally, and spiritually.

*   *   *

"Why me?" I wonder. Why was I spared? With 450,000
people dying of cancer each year, why was I saved from the
grip of death? Why was I given a second chance? Why was
I chosen to live?

"Why me?" Why was I led to macrobiotics? Why did I
put my faith in God and in nature? Why did I believe in the
body's marvelous self-protective and recuperative powers?
Why did I recover?

"Why me?" So many others have succumbed. Good
people, righteous people, giving and caring people, people as
worthy, or more so, than I. Why was I chosen?

I don't know, "Why me?" What I do know is that I am
thankful for my life, for the food that has healed me and
continues to keep me well, for the lessons that my experiences have taught me. I know that I want to give back, to
reach out to others, to teach, to encourage, to inspire, and

to offer hope to those who may be suffering. I want to help people, to spare them the anguish and the agonies that I suffered, to share the experience of a macrobiotic recovery, to offer an alternative to degenerative disease.

I have started by writing this book.

Note to the Reader

Further information on the macrobiotic approach to health can be obtained from The East West Foundation, a non-profit institution established in 1972. The East West Foundation, its major affiliates, and regional offices around the country, offer ongoing classes for the general public in macrobiotic cooking and related subjects.

BOSTON HEADQUARTERS:
Macrobiotics International and
The East West Foundation
17 Station St.
Brookline, MA 02147
(617) 731–0564

MARYLAND
604 East Jappa Road
Towson, MD 21204
(301) 321–4474

CALIFORNIA
1864 Pandora Ave.
W. Los Angeles, CA 90025
(213) 474–2708

COLORADO
1931 Mapleton Ave.
Boulder, CO 80302
(303) 449–6754

CONNECTICUT
98 Washington St.
Middletown, CT 06457
(203) 344–0090

ILLINOIS
5044 North Western Ave.
Chicago, IL 60625
(312) 561–8023

PHILADELPHIA
606 S. Ninth St.
Philadelphia, PA 19147
(215) 922–4567

NEW YORK
32 West 89th Street
New York, NY 10024
(212) 877–1110

FLORIDA
3291 Franklin Ave.
Coconut Grove (Miami),
FL 33133
(305) 448–6625